# CANCER—YOUR LIFE

A compassionate and practical gu...
with this traumatic e...

*In the same series*
AGORAPHOBIA
BEHIND CLOSED DOORS
CARE FOR THE CARER
COPING WITH BEREAVEMENT
COPING WITH BULIMIA
COPING WITH SUDDEN HAIR LOSS
DEMENTIA
EPILEPSY
HELP FOR VICTIMS OF CRIME AND VIOLENCE
HOME IS WHERE THE HURT IS
I CAN'T FACE TOMORROW
LIVING WHILE DYING
LIVING WITH A COLOSTOMY
LIVING WITH TINNITUS
MASTECTOMY
OVERCOMING ADDICTIONS
OVERCOMING ALCOHOLISM
OVERCOMING DEPRESSION
OVERCOMING INFERTILITY
OVERCOMING URINARY INCONTINENCE
QUIT COMPULSIVE GAMBLING
SCHIZOPHRENIA
STEP-PARENTING

# CANCER YOUR LIFE, YOUR CHOICE

## RACHAEL CLYNE

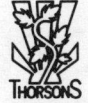

THORSONS PUBLISHING GROUP

First published 1986 as *Coping With Cancer*
This revised edition published 1989

© RACHAEL CLYNE 1986, 1989

*All rights reserved. No part of this book may be reproduced or utilized in any form or by any means, electronic or mechanical, including photocopying, recording or by any information storage and retrieval system, without permission in writing from the Publisher.*

British Library Cataloguing in Publication Data

Clyne, Rachael
Cancer: your life, your choice
1. Man. Cancer. Personal adjustment
I. Title
362.1'96994

ISBN 0-7225-2103-0

*Published by Thorsons Publishers Limited,
Wellingborough, Northamptonshire NN8 2RQ, England*

Printed in Great Britain by Billing & Sons Limited, Worcester

1 3 5 7 9 10 8 6 4 2

This book is dedicated to those whose experience of cancer teaches us all. To those whose courage has taught me that a person is more than the sum of their parts and that Life is definitely an issue of quality rather than quantity.

# ACKNOWLEDGEMENTS

First of all, I want to thank John Hardaker and Thorsons Publishers, without whom I would never have had the opportunity to write this book. Thanks also to Maggie Noach, my literary agent, for her constant encouragement in this my first attempt.

My thanks and gratitude to Roger, for his courage and determination. Although our marriage was brief in years, in learning, its measure cannot be counted. I also wish to thank my sister, Diana, for her love and largeness of spirit. I little realized when I started this book how large a part she would play. Diana tested my beliefs, my ability to love and to 'make sense of it all' in the most powerful way possible. I miss her, but am deeply grateful for the learning and enrichment I have inherited as a consequence. Thanks to Dr Bob Phillips for his willingness to share his warmth and humanity beneath the professional role.

I am grateful to members and associates of CancerLink for their help, with a special thank you to Petra Griffiths for her generous support. I would also like to acknowledge Nola Elbogen for her tireless typing.

Finally I wish to express my deep appreciation for the many members of the Battersea Cancer Support Group, both past and present. Their personal friendship and experiences have taught me much; I hope that through this book they may help many others.

RACHAEL CLYNE

# CONTENTS

Foreword by Petra Griffiths 11
Introduction 13

*Chapter*
1. What is Cancer? — The Medical View 19
2. Diagnosis and Treatment 31
3. Coping With Diagnosis 45
4. Complementary Approaches — The Holistic View 56
5. Mental Attitude 75
6. Relatives and Friends — the Supporters' Experience 90
7. Letting Go 98
8. 'Where Do I Fit Into All This?' 110
9. Patients and Doctors 117
10. Where to Get Help 133
    Appendix: Setting Up a Support Group 139
    Useful Addresses 142
    Recommended Reading 153
    Glossary 156
    Index 159

# FOREWORD

I have followed with delight Rachael's progress in writing *Cancer: your life, your choice* and have looked forward to the day when a book would be available for people going through an experience of cancer that includes all the many ways of being with and responding to the experience.

Having been very disturbed, when I had Hodgkin's disease in 1981, by the separation between orthodox and alternative approaches and oppressed by the weight of the decision as to which approaches to adopt, I would very much have valued having access to a book that presented the various options without foregone conclusions as to which ones are right or best. At the time all the literature I read contained a very definite bias towards particular approaches and very often against others, which added more conflict and tension to what was already a very difficult decision in a life-threatening situation.

*Cancer: your life, your choice* describes both orthodox and complementary methods, not omitting the problems and questions arising with each method. It shows the central place of taking charge of one's life and of one's response to cancer, if one wishes to change the experience from one of fear, powerlessness and negativity, to one that contains also the potential for learning and transformation. Suggestions are given as to how this can be done.

For anyone wishing to take an active approach to a diagnosis of cancer, this book will be an invaluable guide to the many methods available, all of which have been found helpful by some of the people who have trodden this path before.

PETRA GRIFFITHS
Co-founder of CancerLink

# INTRODUCTION

It is quite common for books of this nature to be written as a result of personal experience, and my own case is no exception. Only a few years ago cancer was simply a word which remained on the periphery of my experience; something which happened to other people. The only time it touched me was as a nagging fear whenever I lit a cigarette. Then, within six months of getting married, I found myself flung into the reality when my husband, Roger, was diagnosed with testicular cancer.

Everyone's story has its own drama and intensity; ours was little different, compounded perhaps by the difficulties of a new and somewhat uneasy relationship. When I think back to that period, I find it hard to remember its sequence with accuracy. I remember a jumble of days and weeks, lived at an emotional intensity which now seems impossible to have sustained.

When people talk about 'living each day at a time' as a successful approach to life, I tend to agree with them. At that time, however, I had no choice. Each day seemed to bring at least three impossible decisions to make. Each day the picture changed; results of tests and decisions about treatment which were often delayed, which hospital to use, domestic difficulties, this plan of action, or that plan of action. There was simply no time to think about anything else, like eating or washing, what clothes to wear, or any normal social routine. No time even to think about tomorrow — tomorrow could only be dealt with when it became today.

Fortunately that particular story had a happy ending. My husband's chemotherapy and surgical treatment was successful, combined with his own total commitment to get better and the self-help programme he devised to implement it. He used all sorts of methods to create a positive attitude towards himself and his life, including diet, relaxation, visualization, counselling, etc. For him, it was a much needed opportunity to change the quality of his life to a happier and more fulfilled expression.

He certainly rose to the occasion with courage and single-mindedness determination. Whether or not he would have lived without all this I cannot say, but I have no doubt that he used the situation creatively. He gained infinite benefits from the experience.

After his recovery, we began to look at how our experience might help others. We felt that there was a very definite need to provide something. Although one in four people in Britain gets cancer, at that time (1981) there was remarkably little information or support available to the cancer sufferer. The word 'cancer' alone is enough to make most of us feel distinctly uncomfortable. We still tend to think of it as an immediate death sentence and certainly as incurable. This is despite the fact that many people do recover and others survive for several years.

A large number of people tend to avoid using the word cancer if they can help it and it is still very much an issue whether or not patients are told of their diagnosis. However, the growing demands from individuals who feel they have a right to know and wish to take an active part in their own recovery is helping to change this attitude.

We were very much a part of this movement and in response we set up a cancer support group. In this way we were able to provide basic information about treatment and contacts which patients and relatives needed. We could also offer the opportunity for people to at least talk to someone else who had been through the experience of cancer.

At that time there were only a handful of cancer support groups throughout the UK. Now they are springing up everywhere. There is a slow but growing recognition of their value on the part of the medical profession and in April 1985 the first national conference of cancer support groups was held.

In fact general attitudes to cancer have changed enormously in the last few years. There has been increasing interest in complementary approaches and in the holistic view that cancer is more than just a physical illness and needs to be treated as such. Cancer clinics specializing in complementary therapies are becoming established and have attracted much publicity as a welcome balance to the often drastic treatments used by orthodox medicine.

Some notable advances have been made within the

conventional field, such as with Hodgkin's disease and in the area of child cancer. Whereas ten years ago children were rarely treated at all, many are now treated with success.

Most of us tend to think of cancer as a single disease, when in fact it is the name for a group of over a hundred different diseases, each with its own distinct characteristics. Each person's diagnosis, prognosis and response to treatment can vary tremendously. This has led to the need for people to be considered individually with carefully worked out regimes of treatment. This echoes more and more the holistic view that a patient needs to be treated as an individual rather than as a disease.

There has been a great deal of scepticism and scorn expressed by some of the medical profession when it comes to complementary approaches such as homoeopathy, diet and psycho-spiritual therapies. Non-medical practitioners have been seen as dangerous quacks. Equally, many alternative practitioners have passed judgement on doctors, regarding them as 'bigoted butchers'. It would seem that the two approaches have much to offer each other. Perhaps it is just a reflection of the stage we have reached in a process of change that seems to be taking place within the whole field of health and our attitudes to it. In a sense cancer is a very exciting field to be involved with, as it seems to be on the front-line of all these changes. However, we perhaps need to remind ourselves who we are learning from, for patients are often stuck in the middle with little support or information to help them choose how best to respond to their own disease.

The use of technology in the detection and treatment of cancer has become more and more sophisticated. Patients are often overwhelmed at first by the range of tests and equipment they have to face. Later on they begin to sound like mini-experts when talking about their treatment. However, this emphasis on technology and sophisticated treatment on the physical level has left the patient rather marooned when it comes to emotional support.

Opinions may vary as to the significance of emotional and psychological factors in the disease but the fact remains that the person is facing a life crisis situation with a lot of decisions to make in a short space of time. They have to adjust to a future perhaps permanently uncertain and they need support to cope with this.

One of the most immediate problems which needs to be and is being tackled is the fear we have of cancer and our reluctance to discuss it. Cancer patients often feel so isolated. They may even find that some of their friends back away and appear unsympathetic as they are confronted with their own fear of the disease. Another major problem is the uncertainty with respect to survival rate and recurrence. One doctor in his research has described cancer as a chronic disease which is treated as an acute one.

It is easy for a person to feel isolated and very much the victim of the situation. Whether one agrees with the holistic view that a person is the source and creator of their own 'dis-ease' or with the view that the disease is due to biological factors outside one's control, a positive fighting spirit and enhancement of a sense of well-being are seen by all as very important factors towards survival.

To conclude my own story, the experience of cancer which I have shared with so many has taught me more than I can say. Although I have since parted from my husband, I know that our time together was a tremendous educational experience for us both. Perhaps in its action-packed intensity we completed what we could learn and offer together. I have since begun to learn and develop skills which I personally find helpful to people in all kinds of situations. I have completed a training in psychotherapy and now work as a healer and psychotherapist. My experiences have opened up a whole new life and have offered me an opportunity to fulfil and contribute in a way I never expected.

Cancer, after all, is little different to any life crisis situation. At times, when our survival or the circumstances of our life seem threatened, we often find our priorities changing. Within every crisis, there lies a challenge to discover an opportunity for learning and to gain something of value, however small.

Meanwhile, cancer continues to touch my life, as it touches us all, unexpectedly. While writing this book, my sister was diagnosed with a malignancy. Although of an entirely different nature to Roger, her attitude and faith in many ways was built on the shoulders of his experience. In her own way, she too discovered creative ways to use her predicament.

I hope that this book offers something of that possibility to anyone who may read it, whatever their point of view or opinion. While I recognize that I have taken a personal stance of positivity, I do not underestimate the many difficulties involved. Coping with cancer is by no means easy and frequently involves pain, fear and a great deal of courage.

I hope that my approach does not diminish the challenge confronted by so many, but in the face of that challenge, I feel it is of value. I have attempted to describe the full range of treatments which people are currently using, both orthodox and complementary. I have also given some explanation of the principles on which they are based. I have endeavoured to do this as accurately as possible and without over-colouring the information with my personal opinion. Both choice and opinion are best left to the individual reader.

Meanwhile I hope that whether you are a patient or relative, the personal experiences shared throughout will help to ease any feelings of isolation or fear and show that there is something you and I can do.

# 1.

# WHAT IS CANCER? — THE MEDICAL VIEW

The human body is made up of millions of cells which are constantly growing and dividing to replace old tissue and maintain the body structure. Each organ or type of tissue is composed of cells which are specifically shaped and designed for that location. For example, muscle cells have a very different shape and function to breast or stomach cells.

There is a controlling mechanism which ensures that the new cells are the right shape and that they are reproduced at a rate which does not exceed the needs of that particular body tissue. This means that in an adult, cell birth is roughly equal to cell death.

The information governing cell growth and function is contained in the genetic material or DNA of each cell. This mechanism is also networked throughout the body system. In cancer patients, something goes wrong with the mechanism and certain body cells may start to divide in an uncontrolled and haphazard way. The cells are abnormal in shape and reproduce more rapidly than is needed. If the rate of growth is more than the body can cope with, a tumour or lump begins to form.

**The Difference Between Malignant and Benign Tumours**
A tumour or cyst is not always cancerous and this type is known as *benign*. A benign cyst can increase in size and cause problems which may require its removal by surgery, such as in the case of ovarian cysts. The major difference between a benign tumour and a cancerous or *malignant* one is that it does not spread to other parts of the body. The cells stay in one place and the cyst is often enclosed in a skin or cuticle.

With cancer, the cells tend to break off and invade neighbouring areas. They can get into the blood-stream or lymphatic system, travelling quite a distance from the original or *primary* site. They then begin to form what are commonly called *secondary* tumours. These secondary tumours are medically described as *metastases*. It is this tendency to spread which makes cancer so dangerous.

## Common Types of Cancer and Their Occurrence

There are, as mentioned in the Introduction, over one hundred different types of cancer, each having its own location, characteristics and ways of spreading. For example, breast cancers tend to spread through the lymphatic system affecting the lymph glands under the arm and if unchecked will eventually reach the bone marrow, forming what are commonly known as bone secondaries.

Medical terminology divides cancer into four main groups according to their location and you might find it helpful to know these terms.

**Carcinoma** is by far the commonest group of cancers. These cancers develop in the lining layers of organs such as glands, the lungs, the digestive tract and the skin.

**Sarcoma** is the name given to cancers which arise in the body's supporting tissue (bone, cartilage and muscle) and is much rarer. People may be familiar with the term bone secondaries; this is not the same as bone cancer and refers to secondary spread of malignant growth which develops in the marrow and not in bone tissue itself.

**Leukaemia** describes cancers which affect the blood.

**Lymphomas** —cancers affecting the lymph system.

In Europe and North America, the commonest types of cancer are lung, prostate and bowel cancer in men and breast, uterus and bowel cancer in women. Leukaemia is the commonest form of cancer in children, although childhood cancer is relatively rare. In young adults, Hodgkin's disease and testicular cancer are the most prevalent.

Although people of all ages get cancer, the number of cases increases with age. For breast cancer the peak period is between fifty-five to sixty-five years old. It often seems that the incidence of cancer has increased in recent years but this is hard to assess when other factors are taken into consideration. People live longer and many more cases of cancer are detected and treated than before. We are also much more aware of and willing to discuss the subject.

Chris Williams (a consultant physician and lecturer) states in his highly informative book *All About Cancer* (John Wiley and Sons, 1983), that cancer has not really increased in the last fifty years. What does seem to be true is that some types of cancer have increased whilst others have become less common. The number of lung cancer cases has increased sharply over the last twenty years whereas the incidence of stomach cancer has declined.

## Causes of Cancer

Although cancer is one of the most common diseases (affecting one in four people in this country), it is also one of the most complex. It is therefore difficult to generalize and impossible to speak of in terms of a single cause. Over the years people have hoped that the researchers would come up with 'a universal cure' but we now realize that this is unlikely.

There are still many misconceptions about cancer and how it is caused. Although it is not a contagious disease many people are afraid to go near a cancer patient in case they 'catch it'. In 1973 an interesting survey was done in Lancaster listing popular beliefs about causes of cancer. I have indicated the accuracy of these beliefs in brackets.

| | | |
|---|---|---|
| Smoking | 70 | |
| Not keeping clean | 24 | (There may be a link between a lack of sexual hygiene and the transmission of cervical cancer.) |
| Bad living | 27 | (Not generally true, although there is some coincidence that women who begin sexual relationships at an early age and who have several partners may be prone to cervical cancer.) |
| Contraception | — | (There is evidence to show a link between the Pill and cancer.) |
| Living with people who have it | 7 | (Not true.) |

| | |
|---|---|
| Heredity | 31 (Cancer does seem to run in some families, but only one or two very rare cancers have been found to be hereditary.) |
| Cause not known | 79 |

These spontaneous replies were given to the question 'How can cancer be prevented?'
Don't eat burned food.
Stop falling over.
Don't think too much about it.
Keep your blood in good condition.
Don't eat tinned food.

An aspect which I find confusing is how much research seems to change in its opinion. I once asked 'an expert' whether it was true that the Pill caused cancer. I was told current research showed that it wasn't. Only weeks later the newspapers were filled with a report about the risks of taking the Pill and cancer.

Certain linking factors do seem to remain indisputable, such as smoking and lung cancer. Although not all heavy smokers get cancer it is estimated that 90 per cent of lung cancer is linked with smoking and very few cases are found amongst non-smokers. Cases which do occur are usually of a different kind of lung cancer from that found in smokers. Asbestos is another case in point and the lung cancer which results from exposure to certain types of asbestos is called mesothelioma.

What we commonly think of as causes are usually referred to as risk factors and it would seem that cancer results from a combination of these linked together. Broadly speaking, these risk factors can be divided into two main categories — internal (or personal) and environmental.

### Environmental Factors
The following survey shows estimates for causes of cancer deaths in the United States and is applicable to other Western countries.

| | |
|---|---|
| Diet | 35% |
| Tobacco smoke | 30% |
| Infections | 10% |
| Occupational hazards | 4% |
| Pollution | 2% |

| | |
|---|---|
| Medicines and medical procedures | 1% |
| Industrial products and food additives | 1% |

At this stage I would like to point out how varied and indeed misleading statistics can be. In another similar survey which I read, 30 per cent of cancer deaths in men were attributed to diet and lifestyle whereas 60 per cent of cancer deaths in women were linked to the same cause. Statistics are often based on medically proven figures whereas actual figures may well be quite different. Perhaps it is advisable to think of statistics as providing a very general guideline particularly with something as complex and individual as cancer.

In terms of diet it is thought that lack of fibre and high fat content are the main risk factors. These are particularly linked with bowel and breast cancer respectively. In Europe for example, where we eat a lot of meat and less fruit and vegetables, bowel cancer is quite common. In Africa this balance is reversed; the diet is high in fibre and bowel cancer is very rare. Although no firm conclusions exist, some interesting facts have arisen concerning Japanese women and breast cancer. This type of cancer is relatively rare in Japan, yet Japanese women living in the United States begin to show a similar incidence to that of other American women after only one or two generations. It is thought that a change in diet may well be the linking factor.

Most of us are now familiar with the term *carcinogen*. Carcinogens are cancer-producing substances which, either man-made or otherwise, exist in the environment. Carcinogens affect the DNA and although the body may be able to repair any damage, they can create changes which trigger cancer. The most familiar carcinogens are tobacco tar, asbestos and radioactive material. Even excessive exposure to sunrays can cause skin cancer. Light-skinned Europeans are particularly susceptible. Recent years have shown a dramatic increase in cases of malignant melanoma which some experts believe may be connected to the fashionable use of sunbeds. Environmentalists also blame the damage caused by pollution to the ozone layer.

Many chemical substances have been found to be carcinogenic, particularly certain pesticides and chemical food additives such as nitrates used in preserved meats. Some industrial dyes and chemically-produced food colouring substances are also on the list. This information has largely resulted from experimentation with animals and although the risks are said to be much smaller with humans, new products are constantly being checked for carcinogens.

Unfortunately, the dangers of some carcinogens do not make themselves known until many years after exposure. For example, people who have been exposed to asbestos may not develop cancer until up to twenty years later. The list of carcinogens seems to grow and become endless. It is tempting to throw up one's hands in despair at the impossibility of escaping from all these substances in our environment. Perhaps it is well to remember that carcinogens are only a proportion of the risk factors involved and that fear is another.

The various complementary approaches to cancer put much emphasis on a change of diet and the avoidance of chemically-treated foods of any kind. A high-fibre, raw vegetable diet is usually recommended, with the accent on organically grown 'live' foods. (More details about this can be found in Chapter Four). Although orthodox bodies have been highly cautious about this clinically unproven approach, they are beginning to advise people to change to a more 'healthy' wholefood or vegetarian diet.

**Internal Factors**

In terms of what I call internal or personal factors, we are looking at some of the newer areas of research.

At the beginning of this chapter I mentioned the mechanism which controls the growth and function of cells. As yet, we know little about the nature of this mechanism or how it works. Much research is, however, being focused in this area and some scientists are beginning to discover genes which trigger abnormal growth. These are called *oncogenes* (the prefix *onco-* refers to cancer and *oncology* is the study of cancer).

There is some evidence to show that the body also produces cancer-blocking substances. Dr George Todero, a professor of pathology in Washington, has discovered a protein which he calls oncostain. Oncostain appears to block malignant growth, particularly in cases of lung and breast cancer. Dr Todero believes that there may be a natural tumour-blocking substance for every variety of tumour-growing substance.

The latest area of this kind of research is looking into the relationship between different biochemical substances in the growth mechanism and specifically at what happens when the natural co-operation between these substances breaks down.

Some cancers seem to be linked to hormonal imbalances and

patients are treated with either hormones or chemotherapy to inhibit malignant growth. Cancer of the prostate gland, cancer of the ovaries and certain types of breast cancer are examples where hormone treatment may be used to control the rate of secondary spread.

One or two cancers may be linked to a virus. Cancer of the cervix seems to have a connection with the herpes virus which causes genital warts. It is noted that Jewish women seldom get this type of cancer and it may be that male circumcision offers some form of protection. Some research also indicates that women who have sexual intercourse at a relatively early age and who have a number of partners may be more prone to cervical cancer.

There is a highly controversial theory that all of us produce cancer cells which are normally destroyed by the body. This theory relates cancer growth to suppression of the immune system as a result of stress. The immune system is the body's natural defence against disease and is composed of white blood cells and lymphocytes. These destroy invading bacteria and other forms of infection as well as helping to repair damage caused by cuts and bruises.

Under certain conditions, such as moments of stress, the body system undergoes a rapid change. Stress is the name given to events or triggers which activate what is called the 'fight or flight' mechanism. The 'fight or flight' mechanism occurs when a person feels threatened in any way. Adrenalin secretion is increased and heartbeat becomes more rapid. Blood vessels near the skin contract, withdrawing blood to deeper levels and so lowering body temperature. Breathing becomes faster, digestive secretions decrease and the whole body is in a general state of tension. This mechanism stems from fundamental animal survival instinct, but through the development of a much subtler and more sophisticated way of dealing with situations, we no longer act out the 'fight' or the 'flight' and inhibit our response. Under conditions of chronic or prolonged stress it is suggested that the immune system becomes impaired.

Whether or not we are constantly producing cancer cells, there do seem to be some connections between stress and illness. Dr Hans Selye, in the 1920s, did some research on the effects of stress of the body and, in particular, on connections between emotional stress and illness. Doctors at the Washington School of Medicine later developed this work and designed a scale to measure common stressful events such as the loss of a loved one, retirement and even outstanding personal achievement. Their research showed that people with a very high score, showing high-level stress over a twelve month period, tended to develop illnesses, including cancer.

Dr Carl Simonton (an oncologist) and Stephanie Simonton (a psychotherapist) have done much research and have developed a self-help programme based on the theory of stress-related suppression of the immune system. They run a clinic at Fort Worth in Texas, where patients are taught to identify stress patterns and events in their lives. They are also taught to visualize their immune system, in the form of white blood cells, attacking and destroying cancer cells. The Simontons have written a book called *Getting Well Again* (Bantam Books, 1978) which sets out in great detail information about the mind/body connection with cancer. It describes their self-help methods and documents some of the startling results their work has produced. Although the theory itself is much disputed, there seems to be increasing evidence for the links between personality, stress and cancer. Lawrence Le Shan, another American psychologist, spent ten years researching and exploring these factors with over 200 'terminally ill' patients. In his excellent book *You Can Fight For Your Life* (Thorsons, 1984), he details his findings and includes case histories of some of the seventy patients with whom he worked in depth. This approach is, of course, much favoured by those subscribing to the holistic view. According to the Simontons, there is frequently a time factor of twelve to eighteen months between severe stress triggers, such as the death of a loved one, and the occurrence of cancer.

I have personally known several cancer patients where this has been the case. My husband lost his brother approximately two years before his cancer appeared. Another man I know lost his sister only a year prior to getting cancer. A third man lost his business twelve months previous to developing melanoma (a form of skin cancer which produces malignant growth in a mole). Of course we all experience stressful events at some time or another. Many people undergo prolonged periods of stress without having heart attacks or cancer. However, it seems to be the way we handle stress and not just the stress itself.

The view of those who relate stress to cancer is that patients tend to show common psychological and emotional characteristics. The picture of a cancer-prone personality has begun to emerge. Elements include: early childhood rejection by one or both parents; difficulty in expressing emotions of anger, resentment and grief which causes a bottling up of these feelings and a generally low self-opinion. These elements are coupled with severe stress events such as loss of a loved one, or loss of something with which a person feels deeply identified. There is a marked inability to cope with the stress which results in feelings of helplessness and despair. It is at this stage that a trigger for cancer is provided.

Although I am only stating personal opinion, I have noticed many of these elements to be common amongst cancer patients I have met. There is already common agreement on the type of personality which is prone to heart attack and it is possible that a pattern also exists amongst people prone to cancer. I would like to emphasize that we are talking about a tendency. People can become unnecessarily concerned that they might be the type of person who is *bound* to become ill. I met a young man only recently who was terrified and convinced that he might already have cancer, based on the similarity between his life situation and these opinions.

Finally I would like to mention hereditary tendencies. *Cancer is not generally a hereditary disease.* Only two extremely rare forms of cancer have been found to be hereditary; one is a cancer of the eye found in children and the other is a cancer-prone condition of the bowel. Cancer does seem to run in some families however, and doctors sometimes speak in terms of hereditary predisposition or tendency for cancer to occur. Breast cancer comes under this category, but only under certain conditions and it is by no means thought of as inevitable.

## Can Cancer Be Cured?

It must be clear by now how complex and highly individual cancer is — even people with the same kind of cancer may be diagnosed at different stages and may respond differently to the same treatment. Statistics based on case histories do exist, but they are very general in approach. It is the individual who wants to know how he or she stands. I saw one doctor on television who said: 'People don't often realize that it's really a horse race. You can only tell them what's happened to the other ninety-nine. They want to know what's going to happen to them and you don't know!'

Many people are treated for cancer and never get it again. Some people have cancer and later die from entirely different causes. Others have cancer which recurs yet they live for many years. I have also met one or two people whose cancer had advanced to the degree where they were pronounced terminal, yet they have recovered. With *all* cancer patients, there is a general rule for assessing cure. This is called the five-year survival scale and is to do with the time it takes for all the body cells to replace themselves. If, after treatment, a person shows no further recurrence for five years, then they can officially be called a 'cancer survivor'. Until that period of time has passed, all patients are described as being in remission. *Remission* is the term given when there is no cancer present in the body. *Partial remission* means that there is less cancer present than before. However, it should be noted that five years' remission is no guarantee that cancer will not recur.

Doctors are extremely conservative when speaking in terms of cure; however some cancers are treated very successfully and patients are told that they can be cured. This does of course depend on the stage of development when treated. Hodgkin's disease, certain acute forms of childhood leukaemia, many skin cancers, testicular cancer and a very rare form of cancer called choriocarcinoma (which affects the foetal placenta in pregnant women) are amongst those described as curable. I have actually met a woman who was treated for choriocarcinoma and she has since had a normal pregnancy and has given birth to a perfectly healthy baby. My husband, Roger, was successfully treated in 1982 for testicular cancer and so far has had no recurrence. He was told he had a 95 per cent chance of cure despite the fact that it had spread to his lungs and abdomen. At the time, however, the 5 per cent seemed much larger to him than the other ninety-five.

It is the uncertainty about cancer which people find so hard to cope with because we are still so convinced that cancer is inevitably fatal. Doctors never seem to be able to give definite answers and even if treatment is successful there is always concern that it might recur. Perhaps a positive way of looking at it is that because cancer is so individual, you don't have to base your outcome on someone else's bad experience.

## Recognizing Symptoms

The earlier cancer is caught the better the chances of treatment. Although cancer can be difficult to detect, people are made increasingly aware of possible warning signs. It is far better to risk being a nuisance to your doctor and find out it was all a false alarm, than to avoid going to see him with a worrying symptom and delay diagnosis for months. I have met people who put off going to see their doctor as long as a year because they were afraid of getting the answer.

Cancer of the cervix is one form which can be detected at a very early stage and successfully treated under local anaesthetic. Regular smear tests will show up what are known as *pre-cancer cells*. These are abnormal cells which have not yet reached the stage of forming a tumour.

Regular breast examination is another recommended precaution and there are leaflets informing women how to feel for any unusual lump. (For details see Useful Addresses.) Screening by X-ray does exist for the early detection of breast cancer — this is called mammography. Unfortunately finances have not yet permitted many of these early screening units to be opened in this country.

Chest X-rays are available as an early screening method for all serious lung conditions including cancer.

The warning signals that we are advised to watch out for are as follows:

1. A lump or unusual thickening anywhere (with breasts, a change in shape or inversion of the nipple can also be a warning sign).
2. A sore that doesn't heal.
3. Unusual bleeding or discharge.
4. Marked change in colour or size of a wart or mole.
5. Persistent cough or hoarseness or coughing up of blood.
6. Difficulty in swallowing or persistent indigestion.
7. Change in bowel habits or difficulty in passing urine.
8. Sudden and unaccountable weight loss.

These symptoms do not necessarily mean you've got cancer. They may be due to entirely different and harmless causes, but doctors advise that they should be checked.

As this book includes the validity of personal experience as well as information, I felt it might be worthwhile to include the opinions of some cancer patients about why they think they got cancer and what they felt was instrumental in their recovery.

'I had cancer of the eye twenty-eight years ago and I'm still here. I was forty-five when I had my first child, I'm sure that's what brought it on, but I thought, "Who'll look after my little girl if I go?" and I was determined to see her grown up. I did too and I've got grandchildren now.'

'I don't know why I got cancer; like most people, I thought "Why me?" If I subscribed to the stress view, I suppose I could pinpoint it to my infertility problems and ectopic pregnancy, but I don't wholly agree with that.'

'I believe I was a major factor in causing the onset of my disease. When I was diagnosed I was in a very highly paid job, with a lot of responsibilities and I wasn't coping with it, in fact I had just been given a warning by my boss. I also had marriage problems. When I was told I had leukaemia, my reaction was one of relief, I remember thinking, "At least this'll stop people focusing on how badly I'm doing." Cancer was an escape. It was only three years later that I read about all the psychological connections with cancer.

'Recently I went travelling abroad for six months. While I was away, my blood count was normal. I think this is because I was happy, outgoing and I completely forgot I was a cancer patient.'

# 2.

# DIAGNOSIS AND TREATMENT

Because of the nature of cancer, diagnosis can be quite complicated and can involve several tests before a course of treatment is able to be determined. The type of cancer, exact size of tumour and extent of any spreading all have to be assessed if the treatment is to be successful.

This can be daunting for people as they meet with the range of weird and wonderful equipment which is used. Obviously, it is also a time of anxious waiting before you are able to get any firm answers. If you suspect that you have cancer, every waiting day can feel like a precious day wasted before any action begins; but doctors, like lawyers, are not going to commit themselves until they have firm evidence.

## Who's Who in Treating You?

Knowing which doctor does what and who to ask which question can be confusing for any hospital patient. When you are lying on your back in a strange bed, as well as being in a vulnerable position healthwise, you are totally dependent on the doctors for all information relating to your own condition. You may be seen by various doctors all with different titles, but to you they are just doctors. Visits are frequently brief and for many people it takes some courage and determination to ask all the questions they want and to make sure they are fully answered.

As mentioned previously, you will be looked after by a team of doctors, usually led by a consultant. This is partly because of the combination of methods used in cancer care and partly because of the various grades of doctors which exist within the hospital hierarchy. I thought it might be useful at this point to provide a guide to the different doctors you may encounter and their range of experience and authority.

*House Officer or Houseman:* This doctor is usually in charge of admission and represents the bottom rung of the medical ladder. He or she is described as being pre-registration if out of medical school for less than a year and post-registration after that.

A *Senior Houseman* has more experience.

*Registrar:* This title represents the first step towards specialist training in a particular field of medicine and a doctor may remain at this grade for many years. Registrars usually work as close assistants to the consultant.

A *Senior Registrar* is a very experienced individual. Consultancy posts can be hard to come by and a doctor may remain a senior registrar for his or her medical career despite the fact that he or she may be even more experienced than some consultants.

*Consultant:* The top of the medical ladder. A consultant will have an additional title which describes his or her field of specialization (consultant gynaecologist, consultant oncologist, etc.).

A *Senior Consultant* has even more responsibilities. The chief of chiefs.

*Surgeon:* A doctor who is also a surgeon is usually addressed as Mr or Miss in this country. Surgeons acquire this title once they have passed the second part of their surgical examinations. This antiquated form of differentiation stems from the fact that hundreds of years ago surgeons were not medically recognized and were frequently barbers by profession.

*Physician:* This person is a doctor of internal medicine and is not a surgeon (in the United States, he or she is called an *internist* and physician is the general title given to all doctors).

*Oncologist:* This is a doctor who specializes in the treatment of cancer. Dependent upon the facilities at the hospital where you are being treated, your team may well be headed by a consultant oncologist. An oncologist is usually in charge of chemotherapy treatment.

*Radiotherapist:* This is a doctor who specializes in the field of radiotherapy. It is frequently a radiotherapist who will lead the team caring for you.

*Haematologist:* A specialist in disorders of the blood.

Of all of these doctors it is likely to be the registrar who has the responsibility for supervising your day to day care. Housemen are also frequently the ones to come to your bedside and they will refer any necessary information to the other doctors.

All of these doctors tend to give varying amounts of information. To be fair, doctors also find that patients tend to give differing amounts of information to each doctor, often holding back on facts and feelings which they reserve for the consultant's ears alone.

In addition to the doctors, some hospitals now have specialist nurses who are trained and highly experienced in a particular field of cancer care. They can be an invaluable source of information and emotional support for the patient. One example is the *radiotherapy nurse* who can answer patients' questions about their treatment and give advice on how to cope. The *chemotherapy nurse* often administers the drugs to the patient and is able to give advice and answer questions.

The *mastectomy nurse* advises patients who are going to have this particular type of surgery. She will normally see patients before their operation, answering any questions and helping them to adjust to the prospects of having a mastectomy. After the operation she will arrange to have you fitted with a *prosthesis* (false breast) if that is what you wish and she can advise on any practical problems which may arise. She may also put you in touch with other similar patients if you feel it would be useful to talk to them, or with the *Breast Care And Mastectomy Association*, a volunteer organization which provides the same service.

*Stoma-care* is another area where specialist nurses are available to give support and practical advice to patients. A stoma operation is one which necessitates the removal of part of the lower intestine or bladder. The remaining portion is then diverted to the body surface and an external bag is worn in order to dispose of bodily waste. This may be temporary or permanent. Adjustment to this particular type of operation is often difficult and the *stoma-care nurse* is of invaluable service in helping people to adjust. The mastectomy and stoma-care nurses provide a necessary link in aftercare and continue to be available for as long as they are needed.

The Royal Marsden Cancer Hospital now has a Nutrition department with a qualified dietician, and patients are advised on diet and nutrition during treatment. This is partly to help patients cope with any side-effects from treatments and also in response to the current interest in dietary links with cancer.

## Methods of Diagnosing Cancer

### 1. Biopsy

A biopsy is the name given to the most common method used to identify cancer. It is in fact the only way that cancer can be accurately diagnosed. A small piece of the suspect tissue is removed either by a simple operation or by needle and is sent to the pathology department to be examined. By looking at the cells, pathologists can tell if it is cancer, what type it is and where it has come from. Occasionally the cells are of secondary spread and although they are abnormal in shape, enough information exists to identify their original location. A few types of cancer are difficult to detect even from biopsy and several tests may be needed.

### 2. Radiology

Radiology or X-ray photography is used to show up any suspicious tumour or lump. It can also be used to assess the spread of disease (this is called *staging*). These tests may be done via straightforward photography such as in chest X-ray, or they may involve more complicated methods, such as the injection of dyes to show up areas not normally seen by an X-ray. These tests can be unpleasant but are invaluable as an accurate way of assessing the extent of any spread. *Barium meal* is perhaps the most commonly known and involves swallowing some unpleasant, thick, white liquid which shows up the stomach and intestines. Barium enemas are used for examination of the bowel.

As mentioned previously, cancer frequently spreads through the lymphatic system. This is a transport system of ducts and glands which runs parallel to the blood system. Lymph cells (lymphocytes) and lymph fluid play a major part in the body's immune system, destroying and draining off infection. Most of us are familiar with swollen glands which indicate the activity of a lymph node in fighting infection. Lymph nodes, which act as filters, become enlarged as cancer spreads through them. By injecting a bluish dye through the feet, a large part of the lymph system can be viewed by X-ray. This test is a *lymphangiogram*.

Yet another common test is an IVP (intravenous pyelogram). This shows up the urinary tract (kidneys, ureters, and bladder).

### 3. Scans

Another type of diagnostic test is known as a scan. You may have heard of body scanners or *CAT scans* (CAT stands for Computerized Axial Tomography). This equipment is very expensive but accurate in detecting the presence and spread of cancer. Although not all hospitals in this country have scanning equipment, there are public campaigns which are endeavouring to raise money for their installation. A CT or CAT scan can potentially enable the whole body to be examined. The machine can rotate around the patient and by photographing numerous cross sections of the body, a three-dimensional picture is built up.

There are also other forms of scans which involve either swallowing or being injected with tiny quantities of radioactive material (isotopes). Different types of material are used to show up specific areas. Liver scans, bone scans and kidney scans are done in this way. The radioactivity lasts only for the duration of the examination and so it is not harmful.

Ultrasound is another type of scan for the detection of cancer. This method is based on the same technique as the sonar used by submarines and uses high frequency sound-waves which are bounced through the body. The sound patterns made by the echoes can be analysed and translated into a picture of the area under examination. The advantage of ultrasound is that it is not thought to be dangerous to human tissue but, although it can show up a precise lump, it does not indicate the nature of that lump.

Magnetic resonance imaging (MRI) is one of the latest aids to cancer diagnosis and is particularly useful for viewing the brain, spine and surrounding areas. Without the invasive use of injections or tablets it harnesses the body's own hydrogen molecules to create a picture. These molecules are attracted by the magnetic field of the scanner to form a pattern which can be repeatedly recorded from different positions in order to build up a highly accurate multidimensional picture. MRI is completely painless and also used in detecting the extent of head injuries.

## 4. Blood tests

Having a blood sample taken for examination is relatively simple for the patient but unfortunately it alone does not give enough information to diagnose cancer. Leukaemia is of course one type of cancer where a blood test is important and it is also used in investigating secondary spread in the blood-stream. A few tumours do, however, produce special proteins which appear in the blood. These are called *markers* and by monitoring their presence through regular blood testing, doctors are able to tell at a very early stage if there is any recurrence. Testicular cancer is one type which can be monitored in this way.

## Treatment

There are three major methods used in hospital treatment of cancer: surgery which consists of removing diseased tissue, radiotherapy, and chemotherapy. The basic principle of both radiotherapy and chemotherapy is the destruction of rapidly dividing cells. Treatment invariably includes a combination of these methods and has to be carefully worked out for each individual by a team of different doctors. Surgery is frequently followed up with one of the other therapies to 'mop up' or prevent any spreading. A few cancers can be treated with radiotherapy alone; one example is skin cancer which is successfully treated this way.

Treatment for cancer is often arduous, debilitating and includes unpleasant side-effects. It would be foolish to pretend that this is not so. These side-effects, however, do vary enormously with each individual and according to the type of treatment being given. A positive attitude can make a great deal of difference to a person's experience of his or her treatment and many find that it will actually help to decrease some of the symptoms. You will find more about this approach in the chapter on Mental Attitude which shows how 'accepting' and 'choosing' the treatment has helped some people in this way. Those who allow themselves to sit around and get despondent may only find it harder to cope.

Some people appear to be quite fit when first diagnosed and it can be disconcerting to undergo a treatment which actually makes them feel worse. I think it is important to be aware of side-effects not only from an information point of view but also because many patients become worried about the symptoms they experience during treatment and think that it is the cancer spreading. I have therefore included some of these details. You should have plenty of opportunity to discuss your treatment with the doctor but it helps to know in advance what sort of questions to ask. If you are really interested in obtaining fuller information Chris Williams' book *All About Cancer* gives specific details of tests and individual regimes of treatment for most types of cancer. I should point out however that he includes the general outlook, or prognosis, for each type of cancer, which some of you may feel you do not wish to read.

## 1. Surgery

This is the form of treatment most frequently used. It is essential to remove all the cancerous growth and surgeons will include a surrounding safety margin of healthy tissue to prevent further spreading. Depending on the type and location of the cancer, nearby lymph nodes are often removed as a precautionary measure.

If the growth is small, surgery will be relatively simple. In the case of breast cancer the recent trend is simply to remove the lump (*lumpectomy*) rather than the whole breast (*mastectomy*). Some doctors now feel that a lumpectomy is just as effective as mastectomy and is obviously far less traumatic for a patient. France is a country where this has been become standard practice but in the UK the policy still varies from hospital to hospital and from doctor to doctor. Of course, this will depend very much on the stage of development; if the malignancy is widespread then there is little alternative. Sometimes doctors will advise a woman to have a mastectomy if there is recurrence of malignant growth. If you have had a lumpectomy then your doctor will insist upon a follow-up course of radiotherapy.

## 2. Radiotherapy

Radiotherapy is used to destroy cancer cells by bombarding them with a concentrated beam of X-rays. This is usually done as a course of daily treatments over a period of several weeks — each treatment only lasting a matter of minutes.

One of the main reasons for giving several small doses is to protect the healthy tissues surrounding the area being treated. Radiation affects both normal and cancerous cells. The art of radiotherapy is to destroy the malignant cells completely whilst keeping any other damage to a minimum. The normal cells should be able to replace themselves and the side-effects which people may have during radiotherapy are thought to be far outweighed by its effectiveness as a form of anti-cancer treatment.

Treatment has to be planned individually and with great precision. A patient's first visit to the radiotherapy department is spent planning the course of treatment. Various tests and X-rays will be taken to define the exact area of treatment. The area is then outlined on the skin with a semi-permanent tattoo ink and calculations are made to work out the exact dosage needed.

Radiotherapy is used in three ways:

(a) As a means of destroying or shrinking a tumour (e.g. skin cancer). This is generally at an early stage of disease.
(b) As an addition to surgery. This is to destroy any localized secondary growth and often involves treatment of neighbouring lymph nodes (e.g. breast cancer).
(c) As a palliative treatment. This means that it is used to ease or slow down symptoms rather than cure and is done when cancer has reached an advanced stage. It seemed a strange idea to me when I first heard that radiotherapy could be used to relieve pain, but bone secondaries are often treated in this way.

*Side-effects*

Although the treatment itself is completely painless, most people do experience side-effects during radiotherapy which vary from person to person and according to the area being treated.

Many people associate radiotherapy with hair loss *but this is only so if the head itself is being treated* and only on the area of the scalp under treatment. Any loss of hair is temporary and normal growth begins to return once the treatment is finished. Radiotherapy is only effective as a localized form of treatment; if the cancer is widespread then chemotherapy is generally used. This means that any side-effects are usually localized too. If the lower abdomen is being treated then bowel movements will be affected and patients may have diarrhoea. If the reproductive organs are being treated then infertility can result. With radiotherapy to the head or neck, patients tend to experience loss of taste and a drying up of the salivary glands. This can cause considerable discomfort when eating. General symptoms usually include reddening of the skin on the treated area and tiredness. Again this varies according to the individual, some people are able to continue working although they may find that their energy begins to lapse as the course progresses.

Patients should be given help and advice about coping with any side-effects. Some symptoms are agitated by particular foods and if you are having radiotherapy most hospitals should supply you with a special diet sheet which will help you. At the end of this chapter are some general suggestions which you may find useful.

Another frequent misunderstanding is that the treatment will make you radioactive. This is not so and it is prefectly safe for you to be with other people.

## 3. Implants
There is another form of radiotherapy which involves placing tiny radioactive sources such as beads, wires or needles inside the body. These are placed at the site being treated. Patients are kept in hospital during this treatment which generally lasts for a few days. Because the implant is radioactive, patients are kept in isolation but once the implant is removed and you are discharged there is no longer any risk of contamination. I have met three people who have had this type of treatment, all with different types of cancer. Side-effects vary according to the area under treatment and you should make sure that you discuss this fully with your radiotherapist.

## 4. Laser Therapy
The use of laser beams as a surgical device is becoming increasingly available in the fight against cancer of the cervix. It is possible to detect abnormalities in cervical cells long before they reach the stage of developing into the full blown disease. Treatment involves only a local anaesthetic. A fine laser beam is then directed at the areas of the cervix in question and the cells are burned away. The only thing a woman may notice is a slight burning smell as the laser is operated. Afterwards it is common to have a little bleeding and discharge like a light period.

## 5. Chemotherapy
Chemotherapy or drug treatment is a more recent development in cancer care. Its discovery, however, has some curious connections and dates back to the First World War when a French doctor made some interesting observations concerning the blood cells of mustard gas victims. He noticed that the blood count was lower and the quantity of certain blood cells dramatically reduced. The idea of killing off cancer cells with drugs developed from this. Mustine is the name of one of the chemotherapy drugs derived from mustard gas and is still used today. Many other anti-cancer drugs have since been discovered and new ones are being developed all the time.

All chemotherapy drugs are *cytotoxic* which means that they are poisonous to cells. They affect all rapidly dividing cells and the principle of chemotherapy is that the cancer cells will be completely destroyed whereas normal tissue will be able to replace itself and repair any damage. As with radiotherapy, the treatment is very carefully worked out and the risks involved are weighed against its chances of success as a means of cure.

Chemotherapy has the advantage of treating the whole body system rather than one local area and is generally used when cancer is more widespread. A few cancers can be treated with chemotherapy alone. Several childhood cancers, particularly acute leukaemia, can be successfully treated in this way. Adult cancers which respond well to chemotherapy include Hodgkin's disease and other lymphomas (cancers of the lymphatic system) and teratoma (a testicular cancer). There are also some cancers which do not respond very well to this form of treatment; notably cancers of the digestive system, brain cancer, melanoma and some lung cancers.

Chemotherapy is given in three different ways:

(a) By mouth in tablet form.
(b) By injection.
(c) By intravenous drip.

Although a single drug may be used in some cases, patients are usually given a combination of different drugs. The form of treatment and combination of drugs used vary enormously with each type of cancer.

Some treatments involve a regular stay in hospital over a period of weeks whilst others do not. With testicular cancer, the treatment usually involves a five-day intravenous course every three weeks. My husband had four courses of this type of chemotherapy and was then reassessed. In his case a second operation was necessary to remove the remains of a tumour in the abdomen and no further treatment was needed.

Other chemotherapy courses may involve a single injection or a series of injections every two to three weeks. Some people are given chemotherapy in tablet form and attend as out-patients for frequent checks on their progress.

Chemotherapy is frequently a follow-up to surgery as a means of dealing with secondary growth. As with radiotherapy it can also be used as a means to prolong life rather than cure. As a palliative treatment it will ease or slow down the symptoms, giving what is called prolonged remission. This is in cases where cure is not yet possible or where cancer has reached an advanced stage. Chronic forms of leukaemia can sometimes be controlled in this way.

## Side-effects
Again these will vary from person to person and according to

the particular drugs you are taking. Some people experience few symptoms whilst others are more affected. Your doctor will discuss these aspects with you and you should make sure that you ask all the questions you want to ask and that you raise any doubts you may have. Nearly all courses include rest periods between drugs to counteract the side-effects of the treatment and a short break in treatment is usually possible if things become particularly difficult. Any side-effects begin to clear up as soon as your treatment stops.

General symptoms include chronic tiredness and lack of energy which tends to increase as the course goes on. Some people are able to continue work whilst others find they need to rest.

Chemotherapy affects the blood cells, and regular blood tests or blood counts are taken. White cell count is decreased, so increasing any chance of infection. It is therefore important to avoid contact with anyone who has a cold or flu etc. Other blood cells called platelets, which help to clot the blood, can also be affected, causing increased tendency to bruising and bleeding of the gums. If blood cells fall below a certain level, patients may be given a transfusion or a break in their treatment to allow the blood to recover.

With some chemotherapy courses, loss of appetite and soreness of the mouth occurs. It is important to take extra care over dental hygiene and patients are advised to use a mouthwash to avoid infection. With certain drugs patients may feel nauseous and vomit *but this is not so in every case* and medication can be given to help this. Eating small and frequent meals is suggested and patients are advised to drink plenty of fluids.

*Some* chemotherapy courses involve *temporary* loss of hair *but many do not have this effect*. Hospitals are endeavouring to develop ways of counteracting this; one ingenious method involves a head cooling device made up of a cap filled with ice cubes. This seems to slow down hair loss. Loss of hair is more upsetting to some people than others and hospitals will provide you with a wig to wear until your hair grows back. People often find that the new growth is softer and curlier than before.

Needless to say, the accumulation of these side-effects can also cause depression but this is directly linked with the treatment and *not*, as many people believe, due to their inability to cope, or to the cancer. Once the treatment is finished this heavy sense of debilitation recedes.

## Monoclonal Antibodies (Magic Bullets)

Attempts are being made all the time to improve the effectiveness of treatments and reduce harmful side-effects. One of these recent developments has been nicknamed the magic bullet. Magic bullets are in fact laboratory-produced antibodies. An antibody is a chemical produced by the body in response to the presence of a 'foreign agent' or infection, known as an antigen. Each antibody is tailor-made to recognize and fit its own specific antigen and latches on to it rather like a key in a lock, so preventing the antigen from spreading infection around the body.

Monoclonal antibodies are highly specific chemicals produced artifically and designed to target and latch onto particular tumour cells. They can also be made radioactive and then if injected into the body can act as a homing device to detect the exact site of a tumour. This becomes an additional aid to accurate testing for cancer.

Research is still underway, but it is possible to attach chemotherapy drugs to these magic bullets and thus give treatment directly to the cancer cells *only*, without harming any other parts of the body.

## Nutrition and Dietary Suggestions for Radiotherapy and Chemotherapy Patients

The following guidelines come from the Nutrition Department at the Royal Marsden Hospital, London, and apply to both radiotherapy and chemotherapy patients. The main difficulties, as far as eating are concerned, are loss of appetite and weight loss. Patients can worry unnecessarily about loss of weight and think that it is a symptom of cancer rather than a temporary side-effect of treatment. Relatives can sometimes become over-anxious and add unnecessary pressure to a patient who has difficulty eating. Worrying can also affect weight loss.

The following suggestions have been found to be most helpful in dealing with eating problems.

1. *Start before your treatment.* Where possible begin to think about your diet and try to build yourself up before your treatment starts. People who are well nourished to start with are more likely to cope well and often experience fewer side-effects, including less nausea.

2. *'Eat little and often'* is the golden rule. Several small snacks throughout the day can be easier to cope with and is a good way

to build yourself up. Fresh yogurts are one suggestion.

3. *Eat early in the day.* Symptoms often increase throughout the day, so eating early in the day can be helpful. A larger breakfast is often a good idea.

4. A small glass of sherry or brandy shortly before a meal can be a good way to stimulate your appetite.

5. Try to avoid fried or fatty foods. Spicy foods or high-fibre foods can be troublesome if treatment involves the lower abdomen or bowel (radiotherapy).

6. If your mouth and throat are affected, avoid dry rough foods like bread, fibrous meats and raw vegetables. Patients often find it easier to eat warm rather than hot food. Drink plenty and add gravy or sauces to your food to moisten it. Soft foods like soups, milk puddings and yogurts can be soothing, particularly when chilled. You can also purée or blend meat and vegetables. Sucking ice cubes made with fruit juices can be helpful if your mouth is very dry. If you have a particularly difficult problem with lack of saliva (as do some radiotherapy patients) then ask your doctor about saliva substitutes which are available.

7. There are many ways to enrich your meals adding extra protein and calories to a light diet.

(a) For proteins add milk, eggs, grated cheese, wheatgerm or yogurt to soups, mashed potato, etc.

*Complan* and *Build-up* are two protein supplement products which can be bought at most chemists. Both products come in several flavours and can be made into a nourishing drink.

(b) For extra calories add butter, grated cheese, honey or mayonnaise to food.

There are some high-calorie supplements which you can buy. *Hycal* or *Fortical* are fruit-flavoured glucose drinks which you can also add to fruit or ice-cream. *Caloreen/Maxijoul* is a powder which can be added to both sweet and savoury foods.

## 6. The Latest Developments

I should say at this point, 'Watch this space!', because modern medicine is constantly exploring new ways of combating cancer and this book will need elastic sides to keep up with them. Cancer is one of the biggest and most highly financed areas of medical research.

One example is *differentiation therapy*; a brand new approach to cancer treatment that has begun to show considerable possibilities. It is a combination of drug therapy and vitamin A derivatives which can control cell behaviour rather than destroying them. It may be able eventually to eradicate some cancers but is mostly used as a controller of symptoms. Recent tests in Italy have shown encouraging results in preventing recurrence of lung cancer. It can also be used in conjunction with radiotherapy and chemotherapy to make them more effective.

# 3.

# COPING WITH DIAGNOSIS

To be told that you have cancer is probably a nightmare that many people have had at one time or another. In fact you could almost say that cancer is one of the great 'bogymen' of our time. Many people are reluctant even to speak the word — it has become so synonymous with fear and death. To receive the news that you have cancer is therefore an enormous shock for most people and it is this period of time when first diagnosed which can be the hardest to cope with.

Obtaining the information that you have cancer hasn't always been straightforward. Traditionally, doctors have been seen as remote authority figures who are reluctant to share information with their patients. On the other hand, people have responded by being 'patient', passively waiting for the doctors to tell them what is happening and rarely questioning their treatment. Although these attitudes are changing a great deal, mainly due to the demands of patients, this conditioning still pervades and many of us are of the opinion that our doctors will not tell us the whole truth.

While we all may want doctors to be more open we cannot expect them to be mind-readers. It is just as much up to you to make it patently clear that you want to know all the facts and to make sure that all your questions are answered. The doctor will often wait for a clear clue from you before disclosing information, and subtle hints may not be enough to convince him that you want to be told something.

Because of the fears that abound, doctors are often concerned about your reaction to a diagnosis of cancer. They may be afraid that the shock could make things worse for some patients, and damage their will to recover. This wish to protect the patient has meant that many people have not been told that they have cancer.

Some have never found out, others have found out only years later and some have had to use initiative and persistence in order to obtain the information. I will always remember one elderly lady who finally had to get a sympathetic nurse to nod or shake her head in answer to the question 'Is it cancer?'

Perhaps some people do not wish to know, and I have met relatives of patients who were convinced that they did the right thing in 'not telling'. The kind of remarks they have expressed are: 'He couldn't cope if he knew'; 'It would only add to her distress', and 'She'd just curl up and wait to die'. Sometimes there seems to be an unspoken agreement in a family where everybody knows the situation but where the patient has made it clear that he or she doesn't want it mentioned and wishes to be supported by having things carry on as normally as possible. This strategy can work both ways: it may help to reinforce a positive attitude but it may also add to the strain by making it impossible to talk things over. It is also possible that the stance of 'protecting the patient' from the associated fears unwittingly increases that fear and makes it more difficult for people to surmount.

More and more people, however, do wish to know the diagnosis, and feel that not only is it their right, but that they can cope better if they know all the facts, no matter how poor the outlook. In recent years people have shown an increasing desire to take some responsibility for their own health and have recognized that it can play a vital part in their chances of recovery.

One very practical way of making sure your questions are answered is to write them down. It can be easy to forget or to be tempted to put off asking in the tense atmosphere of a consultation. Show the doctor that you wish to be a partner in your health care and that you feel that mutual trust and co-operation is important. As much as we complain that doctors act like gods dressed in white coats we cannot expect them to do all the work — they need our help! It is an obvious statement but one well worth remembering, that doctors are human too. They don't know all the answers and can only do their best. To quote one doctor on television: 'I think it should be a partnership, we've got to come down off our pedestals. It is like role playing. It's your body, your life and I'm going to help you to the best of our mutual ability!'

Here are some general questions you might find useful to keep in mind when talking to your doctor:

1. What exactly is the matter with me?
2. How widespread is it?
3. What can be done?
4. What is the purpose of this test, what will it involve and how will I be affected?
5. What exactly will this treatment/operation involve?
6. What side-effects does this treatment/operation have?
7. Are these side-effects temporary or permanent?
8. Are there any alternatives to this operation/method of treatment?
9. Is there anything I can do to help myself?

## Responses to Diagnosis

All too often the whole process happens practically overnight. People may feel relatively well, or think that they are being treated for an entirely different complaint and then for one reason or another they find themselves in a hospital faced with the news that they have cancer and the prospect of immediate treatment.

Apart from coping with the fears of what cancer means to you, your whole life is suddenly turned around; domestic arrangements, work and any future plans are instantly altered. It can take a few days at least to begin to adjust to the new situation and yet it is often in those few days that important decisions have to be made. I think it is well worth making sure that, if possible, you give yourself the time and space to adjust and choose clearly, rather than agreeing on the spot, out of panic.

I have met one or two people who were rushed into a course of treatment after having been bluntly told, 'If you don't have this treatment you'll die!' From the point of view of the doctors this may be so, but you will cope far better if you are clear in your own mind about what is happening and if *you* feel satisfied that the plan of action is the best one for you.

Undergoing an intensive course of treatment or major surgery in a state of panic is only going to make it harder for you to cope, and will add to any feelings of negativity. I will talk more about this in Chapter 5, but it is worth mentioning here for two reasons: firstly, if you can begin with a positive attitude towards your illness your ability to cope and chances of recovery are greatly increased; and secondly, you may want to find out more about the operation or treatment proposed. You may even want to have a second opinion, to which you are quite entitled. You can arrange this through your GP if you wish. Don't be afraid of upsetting the doctors; it is your life and even if you end up sticking to the original course of action, at least you will be satisfied in your own mind.

Sometimes people become dissatisfied with treatment they have been given and at a later stage decide to transfer to another hospital. Different hospitals and doctors have different policies and you may have a strong instinct for or against a particular approach. Attitudes towards hospitals also seem to vary from person to person. One person might sing the praises of a particular hospital, while another will have the reverse opinion. Obviously doctors will tend to support their own method of treating cancer but they may not always have the experience or knowledge to advise on alternative options.

Speaking of alternatives, there are a few people who at this point decide to refuse orthodox treatment and pursue alternative methods. If you do decide to do this you will have to be very clear about your course of action. If possible, see if you can get your doctor or GP to support you. Many doctors will be very reluctant to do so but if they are still willing to give you regular check-ups you can at least monitor your progress. Then if you change your mind at any point you will not have lost that connection.

The reactions that people have to diagnosis vary from extreme fear to acceptance. Deep down inside, many people seem to know what is wrong with them and are not entirely surprised with the news. Others are completely shocked and overwhelmed, and being able to talk to someone can be a great help. Apart from nurses who are very sympathetic and helpful listeners, this is a time when a cancer support group can be invaluable. To be able to talk to someone who has survived cancer and who has experienced the treatment can be an immense relief and reassurance.

Relief is a reaction that some people have experienced when they hear the diagnosis (as in the case of one of the people quoted at the end of the first chapter). Often cancer comes in the middle of a critical period of your life; there may have been personal or career difficulties and cancer at least brings one thing to focus — your own well-being. Other problems seem suddenly less significant and for a time at least they have to be put aside while you are taken care of. Many people experience the relief of being able to put a name to what has been bothering them: they may have felt unwell for some time without knowing why and at last someone has found out what the problem is.

For many it all feels unreal at first, as if it were happening to someone else. It always does, doesn't it — never to you, always someone else? Some people try to deny that they have cancer at all. This is perhaps at the heart of those who unconsciously do not wish to know and who go through their treatment without ever discussing their illness with anyone. On the other hand, it is common for people to experience tremendous feelings of sadness and rage as an expression of the question 'Why me?' These are very natural and sane reactions, so don't be afraid of letting yourself express them as openly as possible. Nurses and doctors are very familiar with this kind of reaction so don't feel that you are being abnormally difficult if you find you are experiencing a lot of emotion. Try to recognize exactly what it is that you feel sad or angry about: Sometimes people unintentionally suppress these feelings and express them indirectly by becoming aggressive and resentful towards others: they blame the doctors and can even turn on family and friends.

Talking to someone is one way of expressing your feelings, writing them down or even drawing the way you feel is another. Some cancer patients have found drawing to be a powerful way of expressing and releasing their feelings. It has nothing to do with artistic talent because as children we have all used drawing as a means of expressing and articulating feelings. There is, in fact, a book of children's drawings compiled by an American doctor and called *There's a Rainbow Behind Every Dark Cloud* (Celestial Arts, 1978). The artists are all children who have cancer and they very eloquently express their experiences of the disease, hospital treatment and even death in the form of simple drawings. An English cancer patient, Jen Duncan, found drawing such a meaningful form of expression and self-learning that she held courses for other cancer patients so that they could develop their own 'creative response to cancer'. My husband, Roger, kept a diary all the way through his hospital treatment and found that particularly helpful.

Just as cancer can come at times of crisis and external stress, it can also come at natural turning points in people's lives; menopause, retirement, etc., and it seems to be a dramatic way of bringing that experience to focus. As irony would have it, while I have been writing these chapters, my sister has been diagnosed with ovarian cancer. She had reached a menopausal stage when her cancer was discovered. Previously she was somewhat reluctant fully to connect cancer with psychological or emotional causes but of her own volition her whole experience has, in a matter of days, become more significant as a trigger for inner change than as a physical illness.

Being a wife and mother has been the most important part of her life and she has experienced a great deal of sadness and sense of loss at its passing away. She has also experienced a great deal of fear about what life might hold for her without that function. At the same time, she has become aware of aspects of her life which she has never allowed herself to develop and has felt sadness and anger about that. Fortunately she has also begun to realize the need and opportunity to develop and express these dormant sides of herself and she feels strongly that her cancer came to tell her this. You could call it cancer with a message.

In her own words: 'It's not the cancer I'm afraid of — it was a warning. I can see that and I've got the message. Now I've got the message I don't need it any more, it's served its purpose.'

I can't say whether this kind of interpretation is so in every case, but I do find it extraordinary to watch two people close to me undergo such a powerful experience of change in the meaning of their lives. For Roger, cancer was also a transformative experience. In the months before his diagnosis it was as if he erupted with years of bottled-up fear and anger. His behaviour became wildly unpredictable and he was physically violent towards me. He couldn't understand why he was acting that way. As a result, we were in the process of splitting up when his cancer was diagnosed. Once he was diagnosed, he seemed to begin to come together and was exceptionally calm and strong-willed in dealing with his illness. In fact, we did part at that time for about two months and he used the separation to look closely at his emotional life. He was able to come to terms with lifelong feelings of resentment and self-hatred. Through the experience of cancer he developed a new faith and confidence in himself. He never seemed to doubt his chances of recovery and developed the ability to take each day as it comes without fear of the future. His cancer seemed to be about learning to love himself and discovering a way to express the uniqueness of his own life.

We often wondered how common these problems of physical aggression and relationship difficulties might be. Once cancer is diagnosed everyone's attention becomes focused on the physical level and perhaps these aspects don't get dealt with or recognized. In our case nobody was sufficiently well-acquainted with the situation to be able to see what was happening or to help. Eventually it did come to the attention of one of the hospital social workers and I found it reassuring and helpful to be able to talk to her. It was only then that I discovered that it was not an unknown experience.

Roger and I once saw a play on television about a man who, after being made redundant, began to act strangely and aggressively towards his wife. Nobody could make sense of his behaviour, then suddenly he was diagnosed with a brain tumour. It was only a play but it was so close to our own experience that we just sat and wept all the way through. It was such a relief to know that we were not the only ones to have had such an experience. Of course, the kind of situation Roger and I went through was an exceptional one, but I felt that it was worth including for the sake of those few who might be experiencing something similar.

For the most part, this is a time when family and friends draw closer together and provide much-needed support for each other. Cancer is certainly something which affects the whole family and if matters can be discussed as openly as possible then all the better. Who to tell and how to break the news is often an issue to be considered, particularly where children are concerned. I have met several people who have felt it important to share the news with their children. Children will usually realize that there is something wrong and often feel safer if they can understand and share in what is happening. One friend of mine was quite open about her mastectomy with her four-year-old son. As many children do, he took it very much in his stride and I know that she has felt much easier at not having to hide things from him. I have also met one or two people who decided not to tell their children and, although they are convinced that they were right, keeping the situation a secret has put a considerable strain on them.

Sometimes people find that they would rather not tell certain friends or relatives, particularly if those people are prone to over-reacting or over-sympathizing. It can be hard enough to cope with your own reactions without having to handle someone else's fear and distress as well.

Don't feel you have to put up with unsupportive company simply because you are afraid of upsetting someone's feelings. It is important that you are surrounded with the kind of love and support that you need. People often find new friendships — acquaintances they scarcely knew before suddenly turn out to be stalwart supporters. Occasionally, people find that a friend who has been close suddenly becomes scarce. It can seem hurtful, but many people are frightened of cancer and some quite simply, have an aversion to hospitals and illness in general. Although it may be disappointing, in a way these friends are supporting you as best they can. If they do feel unduly negative it is perhaps best that they are not around and that they don't add their negativity to the scene.

Unfortunately, a large number of people who get cancer are elderly and live alone. Their friends have gone and their family may live far away. Perhaps for them cancer may be a symptom of their loneliness and often even a hospital can provide a haven of care and company for a while. When I first became involved in setting up the cancer support group, we received many calls from single elderly people who were glad not only of the support but also of the social contact. They were glad too, to be able to offer something useful to others.

If you are alone it can be all the more important to find some kind of support and friendship in your neighbourhood, particularly if you are undergoing lengthy treatment or have had debilitating surgery. Physical comfort is important too. Some people feel as if their body has been taken over by a kind of alien. Cancer is rarely something you can see and yet people can become repulsed by their own body. Loving contact, even if it is only a friendly hug or an arm around your shoulder, can be an immense comfort.

Accepting and loving your body can be very healing. Your poor body is endeavouring to fight the illness and is also taking all kinds of 'bashing' from the treatment it is receiving. Strange as it may seem, some people find that talking to their body is helpful. Taking time to look at yourself in a mirror and touching your own body are other ways to acceptance. If you have had surgery which results in some kind of disfigurement, such as mastectomy, or a stoma operation, then it is all the more important. Learning to adjust and accept your 'new' body can be difficult for some, particularly within a close relationship. Many people are surprised and relieved to find that they are still acceptable to and loved by their partners, but for those who do experience difficulties, communicating them openly with each other is often far more helpful than bottling things up and hoping that they will all go away.

Counselling can be a great help. As mentioned in the last chapter, some hospitals now have specialist nurses who help

## COPING WITH DIAGNOSIS

patients to deal with particular problems. If there is a mastectomy nurse or a stoma care nurse at your hospital, do not hesitate to talk to her about your worries. There are also various organizations which can be useful contacts; The Breast Care And Mastectomy Association and the Colostomy Welfare Group are two such organizations and you will find their addresses at the end of the book. The people who run these associations have all had the particular operation involved and so they will have some understanding of your experience. There is also an organization called *SPOD* (Sexual Problems of the Disabled) to which you can write if you have particular problems in that area. SPOD publishes some helpful leaflets and again I have included the address in the last chapter. Some local health authorities and hospitals now run sexual advice clinics so it is well worth enquiring if you want help. The counselling is always strictly confidential and the advisors are experienced.

### Finances

Finances are often a major consideration because lengthy illness or prolonged treatments can create problems in this area. If you need financial assistance, your hospital or local authority social services department may be able to help. There are also grants available for cancer patients from organizations such as Cancer Relief. They may not be huge amounts of money but can be helpful in covering extra items not included in state benefit, e.g. extra heating costs, bedding, extra travel, etc. Your GP or hospital social worker will apply on your behalf. For parents of children with cancer, The Malcolm Sargent Cancer Fund for Children is another source of extra financial help and again your hospital social worker will apply for you.

If you qualify to be registered as disabled it can be of financial benefit as there are many extra concessions which are available to disabled people. Some local authorities, for example, can arrange for you to go away for convalescence and provide a much needed rest and holiday after hospital treatment.

### Ways of Coping

The majority of cancer patients I have encountered, quickly become avid seekers of information. The recent wave of interest and opening of awareness about cancer has produced a whole rash of books (including this one), networks and experts in the field. It is almost as if patients could enter a university and read for a degree in cancer. However, while the wish to be well informed is a healthy one, it can also have its pitfalls. Some books may be highly informative but they may also evoke unwarranted fear or express a particular opinion which does not necessarily relate to you. The same can apply to talking to other people. We all like to identify with others who seem to be in the same situation as ourselves but, as I have emphasized before, cancer is so individual that what has happened to someone else may not apply to you. Try to select what you need and what you feel will be most helpful to you.

Having cancer seems to require a mixture of courage and acceptance; the will to fight and the patience to accept each day as it comes. The picture is constantly changing, results which were supposed to come today do not arrive till tomorrow or the next day and so on it goes. Morale can be hard to sustain throughout lengthy and often arduous treatment. After a while people may find that the treatment drains them of the energy they need to fight the disease and extra support is valued at this point.

When Roger was receiving chemotherapy, he managed to create around him a very powerful atmosphere of patience and calm. This affected me deeply, there was no future to worry about. By living each moment at a time, I felt everything was OK and was going to be OK, however it turned out. It was very peaceful. We both found a lot of comfort from a card which is published by Alcoholics Anonymous. It is called the *Just for Today* card and it starts:

> Just for today I will try to live through this day only and not tackle my whole life problem at once. I can do something for twelve hours that would appal me if I felt I had to keep it up for a life-time.

It is important to remember that you are still a person and not a walking illness. It is possible to become obsessed with cancer and although it is good to be able to talk about it, it is also good to be able to put it aside too. If you can, try to create some areas of enjoyment in your life, where you can forget about being a cancer patient and focus your attention on some of the qualities of health rather than on the qualities of illness.

The fear of recurrence and coping with recurrence are also problems which have to be faced. Every time you feel under the weather or have a twinge or a headache, there is always that niggling thought that it might be cancer again. If you are concerned, it is always worth consulting your doctor. He or she will be only too happy to be able to put your mind at rest and if there is a cause for that concern, then it can be handled as quickly as possible. As I have already mentioned, people frequently mistake side-effects of treatment for symptoms of cancer. If you have had surgery it will often take more time than you think for your body to recover and repair itself and the resultant aches and pains can cause unnecessary concern.

If cancer does recur, it can be a real blow — all that positive spirit and will to fight seems to have been to no avail. You feel that somehow you thought you'd had it licked and now you've failed, but it doesn't have to mean the end. I know many people who have recovered successfully even after recurrence. Mustering those qualities of courage and acceptance becomes all the more important, the courage to fight and the courage to accept what is. It may be that developing self-acceptance and quality of life becomes more important than physical outcome. Fulfilment doesn't necessarily depend upon length of survival.

Recently I went to hear the Dalai Lama speak. He has endured a very difficult life, exiled from his own country for many years and yet still the acknowledged leader of his people. He is supposed to represent the spirit of compassion and in spite of the difficulties he has had, he remains a remarkably light and humorous man who inspires all who meet him. Someone asked him the question, 'What if you fail?' He replied gently and without hesitation: 'Then you try again and if you fail again, then again you try and you keep on trying, that is all!'

# 4.

# COMPLEMENTARY APPROACHES — THE HOLISTIC VIEW

**Background**
During the last few years there has been a tremendous surge of interest in what is often referred to as alternative medicine. *Complementary* and *holistic* are also terms which are popularly used to describe a whole range of different therapies currently being practised outside the domains of conventional medicine. Some therapies, such as acupuncture, have been practised for well over a thousand years. Others, more recently developed, have grown out of the new movement. All of these therapies are naturally based and involve the use of neither drugs nor surgery. Some treatments, such as herbalism and homoeopathy, involve the taking of natural remedies and others, like osteopathy, may involve subtle manipulation of the body structure.

Perhaps more than any other disease, cancer has become increasingly associated with alternative treatments and the holistic view of illness. At last something new seemed to have come into the picture in the long struggle to beat the dreaded cancer. There is an information and networking organization called New Approaches to Cancer and a growing list of holistic cancer practitioners. Holistic cancer centres are becoming established. The first and most notable of these is the Bristol Cancer Help Centre, whose new clinic was officially opened by HRH Prince Charles in 1983.

Most important of all, there is a growing body of pioneer cancer survivors who attribute their recovery to the holistic or combination approach. This is despite tremendous opposition from the medical profession. Not only have they had to fight cancer but also the prejudice and lack of support of their own doctors. To be fair, most doctors have held their view in what they thought to be their patients' best interests. After all, none of the therapies has been clinically proven and most practitioners are medically unqualified.

However, there is a small but growing number of doctors who have become renegades within their own profession and in 1983 a British Holistic Medical Association was formed, under the focus of Dr Patrick Pietroni from Queen Mary's Hospital, Paddington. As far as pioneering the holistic approach to cancer care in this country is concerned, the two names which spring most readily to mind are Dr Ian Pearce and Dr Alec Forbes. Ian Pearce, author and retired GP, was a trustee of both New Approaches to Cancer and the Bristol centre before his death in 1987. He was a gentle visionary who sought to lend his medical backing to give the new ideas a chance for recognition. Dr Alec Forbes was the founder of the Bristol Cancer Help Centre. His work did much to open up a dialogue between holistic practitioners and members of the medical profession.

Alternative medicine has so far grown in a rather diffuse and unrestricted way. The more established therapies have their own rigorous training before professional status is granted. Acupuncturists, for example, can spend four years in training before gaining qualification. Other therapies are less well established and there is little indication of a practitioner's level of experience — the only recommendation being the word of the client. This has led to a blanket view that practitioners are quacks and charlatans, much to the chagrin of those who are highly qualified and experienced within their own field.

The increasing interest in alternative medicine and the demands of patients have drawn the attention of the British Medical Association. In addition, alternative medicine seems to have won the championship of Prince Charles who astounded the BMA with his inaugural speech as President of the Association in 1982. He urged the medical profession to look beyond the boundaries of man as simply a machine in need of repair and he warned of the risk of overdependency on drugs as a form of treatment. He spoke of the need to see and treat the whole person and encouraged doctors to take more seriously those natural therapies which incorporate that approach. As a result of this challenge the BMA held an investigation into alternative methods of treatment, but found little evidence to change their view.

The difficulty is that we are dealing with two such entirely different models of medicine that it is hard for one to judge the other on its own terms. The orthodox and holistic approaches come from a different philosophical basis or world view so it is not surprising that there is conflict and confusion in seeking to find common ground. It is rather like trying to compare Chinese with English.

Yet there is much they can lend each other; hence the term complementary. Perhaps it is through the many cancer patients who explore diet, healing, and holistic vision in addition to their orthodox treatment that this complement will ultimately be found.

Indeed, it is largely due to the enthusiasm of patients that some alternative practices are finding their way into the medical system in a very small way. There is increasing appreciation of the need for counselling and emotional support even if there is not yet the provision for it. Relaxation and visualization are beginning to be used in a few radiotherapy departments and there is much more awareness of the importance of diet and nutrition. Some doctors have done limited training in therapies such as acupuncture or homoeopathy, although many only use the techniques from their allopathic framework in order to get rid of symptoms rather than treating the whole person.

At present the two systems lie side by side with little real dialogue between them but at least a more open recognition of each other's existence. Perhaps at this stage that is the best we can hope for.

The danger comes when alternative techniques are viewed as useful bits to be tacked onto the established system and orthodox medicine seeks to maintain its control without properly taking into account the true nature of holism or the relevance of its non-medical practitioners.

So far Britain has escaped the kind of restrictions placed on 'fringe' practitioners throughout the rest of Europe and the USA, where non-medically qualified practitioners have to work under the supervision of a doctor. The UK will eventually adopt similar regulations. In the meantime this is forcing the haphazard collection of alternative therapies to bring its house into order and adopt some of the strengths of the orthodox system in terms of cohesion and a proper system of evaluation, and qualification.

One way of looking at the two modes of medicine is in relation to what are called the masculine and feminine principles. In a very limited fashion we use these principles to form our judgements about what is male and what is female but their reality is far larger. The masculine and feminine are universal principles which express whole ranges of qualities and ways of relating to life and they are unlimited by gender. The ancient Chinese coined the term yin and yang and based systems of medicines, diet, aesthetics and even business on creating a harmonious balance between the two.

To return to our two approaches to health, orthodox or allopathic medicine is largely governed by the masculine principle, and holistic medicine is in turn strongly influenced by the feminine.

From the masculine stance reality is viewed through the parts rather than the whole. It is by the logical fitting together of well-defined parts that a satisfying whole is created. The emphasis is on definition, logic, order, and hierachy. Some of the primary strengths of the masculine are detachment, clarity, order, and containment.

From this basis it is easy to see why modern medicine has focused so much on the mechanics of illness and on how the body works. It also explains why it has busied itself on clarifying and distinguishing all the parts and functions from each other in an awesome catalogue of symptoms. Medicine has been brilliant in doing this and has developed superb technology to deal with the mechanics of symptomatic treatment. It is also easy to understand why skills of intellect, reason and objectivity are valued so highly by allopathic practitioners.

The danger is that when this becomes the only view of the universe and an imbalance is created then the whole becomes lost in the parts. Rigid authoritarianism and lack of awareness of other as a living force are negative aspects of the masculine. Control replaces co-operation and medicine starts to be about stamping out or getting rid of symptoms rather than nurturing health. The body manifesting the illness becomes split off from the living being experiencing it and illness becomes a mechanical fault to be corrected rather than an expression of wholeness attempting to rebalance itself.

By contrast, holism, as an expression of the feminine, functions from relationship or connectedness. Holism is a way of perceiving in terms of wholeness. From a holistic point of view, nothing is separate but always part of and reflective of a greater whole. Life becomes an ever flowing process rather than a series of separate events. Illness is seen as a trough of that same continuous wave. Quality becomes more important than quantity and reality is perceived empathetically or subjectively rather than intellectually.

This way of perceiving life is emerging in many fields of knowledge, such as physics, where scientists have given up the search for the smallest particle. In seeing that the field or pattern may be the defining factor, they have also come to the realization that the observer is not separate from the observed. The two may in fact be participating in an act of mutual creation, observer affecting the observed, and that reality only exists in relationship.

Holography, or three-dimensional photography, uses laser beams to project its images. The most startling discovery about holograms is the fact that no matter how many times you split the beam projecting the image, you will always get a picture of the whole image. In other words, the whole image is contained in every particle of the beam. This for me seems to sum it all up and in terms of health you cannot separate the mind, body, feelings and spirit of the individual; they are one organism. *Physical illness is viewed as a symptom of imbalance or a condition which runs through the whole system. Any illness has a correspondent cause and effect on each of the levels of being. As a result, holistic medicine aims to treat the whole person, rather than the physical illness. It endeavours to evoke the person's own natural self-healing capacities in order to restore balance and wholeness.*

In contrast to allopathic medicine the holistic approach therefore concentrates its treatment on strengthening health and the qualities of health rather than destroying symptoms. This is why we associate the new approaches with positive thinking, active well-being, relaxing, and natural foods etc. From a holistic point of view, symptomatic or allopathic medicine often only removes the symptoms without addressing the cause. In viewing things holistically, one is always looking for connecting patterns or qualities that seem to run through the whole system.

Healing the personality, and the stress patterns described in the first chapter, are seen as crucial in dealing with cancer. On the physical level, the focus is on nutrition and replacing stressful and toxic diets. Cancer can be broadly viewed as a result of decreasing co-operation with the natural flow of Life.

Modern diet has moved further and further away from natural foods (often described as *whole*foods). Everything has been processed, forced, added to and the natural quality of our diet has decreased more and more without our noticing quite how far we've let it go. Junk food is a term which adequately describes meals often less nutritious than the packets they come in!

Inner stress has increased as modern living has grown further and further away from a natural environment. Modern times bring other pressures to bear as for the first time we sit with the reality that we could now blow ourselves and the whole planet apart. (Life-threatening illness on a global scale?)

To bring it back to focus, cancer is seen as a whole system illness which needs to be tackled on all levels. The view is that burning, poisoning or cutting out the tumour is not sufficient to cure the illness and that the mind and emotions have to be treated as well if health or wholeness is to occur.

Although there are general patterns, the individual expression of those patterns has to be taken into account. Each person has a different story and a different set of triggers which connect with his or her situation. In other words, it is the person who makes the difference to the illness and two people with similar looking illnesses may have completely different connecting factors. To quote Lawrence Le Shan's excellent book *Holistic Health* (Thorsons, 1984): 'Each sick person is an entire universe with positive and negative forces interacting in very intricate ways.'

The relationship between patient and doctor and the view about 'who's curing who', is frequently different. The emphasis is very much on partnership, with the therapist providing the right environment for the clients to heal themselves. It is thought that you cannot in fact heal somebody else and in the end there is only self healing. This is why there is so much stress on personal responsibility, not as blame, but as an expression of 'this is my illness and I am the source of my own healing.'

For a truly holistic practitioner, it doesn't make sense to categorize people in terms of their illnesses — to generalize about breast cancer patients as opposed to lung cancer patients, or even to talk about cancer patients at all. On the other hand, it can seem just as bizarre to a conventional doctor to relate tumours to repressed anger and attitudes of self-denial and to believe that by resolving these issues, tumours can disappear.

Because of the feminine principle approach and the context of relatedness, the qualities of empathy and intuition are extremely important in a holistic practitioner. It is through these relationship skills as much as observation that practitioners are able to *tune* into the feelings, mind, and body of the person and link the patterns of imbalance together. This is in stark contrast to the professional distance and lack of personal involvement valued by orthodox practitioners. In the face of this it is perhaps easier to understand why the two styles are so sceptical of each other and also perhaps why they are both needed. Both have their limitations. The feminine principle also has its distortions if expressed in an imbalanced way. There can be a lack of objectivity or clarity and a tendency to make assumptions which are not always substantiated.

To sum up: the term 'holistic' refers to a context or way of thinking. Applied to the field of medicine it is an attitude or approach to health and healing, rather than the techniques which may be used. There is a current misconception that unorthodox therapies are 'holistic'. While many may be based upon holistic principles, it is the way they are used which makes them holistic. A practitioner who sees his particular method as the only way is not holistic. A nutritionist who tells you that cancer is caused by dietary deficiencies, which will be cured by his method, is no more holistic than the surgeon whose only answer is to remove the lump.

**Therapies Used in Complementary Approaches to Cancer**
Most people use a combination package of different therapies (e.g. diet, psychotherapy and healing) and in fact this multiple level approach is strongly advised by places like the Bristol Centre. It is thought that one type of therapy on its own is insufficient. I have found, however, that people will often identify with one therapy more than another — there are those who become very involved in the dietary approach while resisting the psychotherapeutic one and vice versa.

In this part of the chapter I have listed some of the more commonly used therapies with a brief explanation of each. Unfortunately there is not enough room in this book to go into full details of all of them and where possible I have listed the appropriate reference books for you to consult.

A. Nutrition and dietary approaches
1. *The raw food diet*
This particular diet has become the best known of all the alternative anti-cancer treatments and it is perhaps the one which has raised the most controversy with the medical profession. Apart from increasing health, one of the main purposes of the raw food diet is to cleanse or detoxify the body and rid it of both cancer cells and the toxins produced by eating a modern junk food diet. If followed completely, it is a stringent diet and for many

it involves a total transformation of personal eating habits. The diet is based on an even more extreme version, called Gerson Therapy. This was developed by a man called Max Gerson who used it with different chronic conditions, including cancer. He is no longer alive, but his therapy is still used.

Basically, one is required to eat plenty of organically-grown raw vegetables and salads. Cooking often destroys valuable nutrients, while raw foods are full of 'life energy' which the body needs. Fruit and freshly extracted fruit juices are also recommended. Freshly-made carrot juice, rich in vitamin A, is thought to be especially important in combating cancer and you are encouraged to drink at least 8 fl oz (230ml/1 cup) per day. The juice has to be emulsified with a few drops of cold-pressed oil to enable it to reach the cancer cells more effectively.

Herb teas, spring water and filtered tap water are allowed. Some cooked food can be included, but must be prepared in a way that is least destructive. Gentle steaming is fine, but fried foods are completely forbidden.

This brings us to the 'don'ts', or the foods to be avoided. For many the list may seem to include virtually all of their present diet. No alcohol, tobacco, tea, coffee, salt or sugar may be taken. This includes the many manufactured foods which contain salt or sugar additives. No meat — factory farmed animals contain high levels of hormones and antibiotics. Processed foods of any kind should be avoided (refined flour, polished rice, etc.). Dairy foods, like milk, cheese and eggs, are also excluded. The belief behind this aspect is that animal proteins use up certain enzymes for their digestion, which could otherwise play an important part in the destruction of cancer cells.

After the first three to six months, patients are allowed to ease up slightly and include items such as freshly-made yogurt or buttermilk and even, very occasionally, white meats like fish and free-range chicken.

Another important component of this diet is the use of naturally produced vitamin and mineral supplements. Vitamin C is thought to be particularly important as it strengthens the immune system and increases vitality. Patients are encouraged to increase their daily dosage gradually to between ten and fifteen grammes.

2. *Macrobiotics*

A less well-known form of nutritional treatment for cancer is the macrobiotic diet. I have, however, known two people who used it successfully without having any orthodox treatment. One woman had breast cancer six years ago and so far has had no recurrence. The second woman had cervical cancer and has been using macrobiotics for two years without any problems.

The concept is based on the oriental principles of yin and yang (feminine/passive and masculine/active energies). It involves a fairly complex system of categorizing different foods according to their yin or yang properties. Root vegetables such as carrots and turnips are more yang, but potatoes and tomatoes, for example, are extremely yin. The idea is to maintain the correct balance of yin and yang in one's diet. Illness is held to be the result of imbalance. Specific macrobiotic diets are used to treat different conditions, including cancer. Anyone interested in using macrobiotics would need an individual consultation for their own specific diet to be worked out.

The cuisine tends to be 'wholefood Japanese' in style; with plenty of brown rice, beancurd (tofu), seaweeds and naturally fermented soya sauce (tamari). As with the raw food diet, chemical additives and processed foods are out. In contrast, however, most of the food is cooked rather than raw. The general diet is composed of 50-60 per cent grains, 20-30 per cent vegetables and occasional amounts of more natural meats such as fish and free-range chicken.

Macrobiotic groups can be found in France, Germany, Portugal and Spain. There are large centres in Belgium, Holland and Boston, USA. In this country the Community Health Foundation and Michio Kushi Institute in London, provides the main centre (see Useful Addresses). Other groups are being set up in Edinburgh, Brighton, Bristol and Leicester.

Diet can become a way of life and can involve an awful lot of food preparation, but many believe the results are worth it. People are advised to move gradually into the raw food diet without changing too drastically overnight. It is important that the diet does not become another source of stress and many advocates are now encouraging patients to aim towards its general principles, rather than following it to the letter.

*As with all holistic treatments it is the quality with which you use it which makes the difference.* I have seen cancer patients who have used diet as a punishment, reinforcing patterns of self-denial, rather than using it as an expression of health and nourishment. People can see the diet as a form of restriction, as a set of rules which have to be kept at all costs. This often leads to feelings of guilt and failure if the 'rules' are broken.

Personally I find the whole area of health food, diet and nutrition a sticky one. There are so many conflicting opinions and beliefs about different foods and vitamins. People seem to enjoy arguing about health foods almost as much as they do about politics. However, it is important to remember that in the centre of this situation is a very vulnerable person. It is easy to fall into the belief that the diet is going to save you. I knew a patient who faithfully followed one diet and then went for a consultation with a proponent of a different system of nutrition. He was told that everything he had been doing was wrong and you can imagine how upset and frightened he became.

It is also important that it is the patient's choice to go on such a regime. I have unfortunately come across two cases where people who did not know that they had cancer were put on raw food diets by their families. You can imagine their feelings of confusion and distress at finding themselves suddenly forced to eat lots of 'strange food'.

Diet can be a valuable tool, providing expression for the people's need to help themselves and their will to recover. It can increase the experience of bodily health and vigour. Many people find they enjoy taking a more active interest in the food they eat and how it affects them — they are taking time to nourish and care for themselves. *Giving oneself nourishment is an emotional and psychological act as well as a physical one.* Many people also begin to develop a natural sensitivity to the foods they need. They are intuitively drawn to some foods and not to others and they are exceptionally aware of the effect different foods have on their body. People usually continue with the basic principles of their diet long after recovery. This is in order to prevent recurrence and also because it has become part of their new outlook on life.

## B. Homoeopathy

Homoeopathy was developed by a German doctor, Samuel Hahnemann, who died in 1843. It uses the immunity principles of treating like with like, and by aggravating the symptoms it provokes the body into producing an immunity. It is a holistic therapy, aiming to treat the person rather than the disease.

Miniscule quantities of the remedies are added to a solution of distilled water and alcohol. Sometimes the amount is so small that it is undetectable. The fact that these remedies work has long puzzled scientists. Critics claimed that they acted as a placebo but this has been disproved by experiments with bacterial cultures which were affected by the remedies.

In this country the Royal Family have long been users of homoeopathy. Their patronage has given it a respectability and protection which has so far evaded the other major therapies and, in fact, homoeopathy is available within the NHS. In London there is a Royal Homoeopathic Hospital which was founded in 1850. There are a number of doctors who practise homoeopathy but there are also many homoeopaths who are medically unqualified.

Homoeopathic treatment of cancer is invariably used as an alternative to conventional methods. However, some people find that certain remedies such as arnica can be very helpful in recovering from the shock of an operation. The remedy which is used to treat cancer is derived from mistletoe and is called iscador. After an initial treatment, patients are taught to inject themselves with iscador on a regular basis. One woman I know has maintained this treatment for nearly five years. Originally she had a lumpectomy but then refused radiotherapy. She combined homoeopathy with the raw food diet, visualization and counselling. She is still free of cancer.

Homoeopathy is practised in the USA and many European countries, particularly France and Germany. India and Pakistan have a flourishing tradition of homoeopathy and many of the Asian GPs who practise in this country have a knowledge of the remedies.

One note of caution — not all doctors practise homoeopathy in a truly holistic way and will use the remedies to get rid of symptoms rather than treating imbalances within the individual.

### C. Stress release techniques.

Relaxation, visualization, meditation and biofeedback training are methods which people use to let go of tension and stress. They are essentially self-healing techniques which can be perceived either as an active anti-cancer therapy or as an aid to coping with the stresses of illness and treatment.

Mind training techniques have been practised in the East for thousands of years, partly as a spiritual discipline and partly for their health benefits. We, in modern western society, have now begun to appreciate the value and enjoyment of developing a quieter mind. Increasing numbers of people are taking up meditation as a daily discipline.

There is no doubt that certain physiological changes occur when the body and mind are in a deeply relaxed state: brain wave rhythms shift to the lower alpha frequencies, muscles relax, heartbeat slows down and the system is generally given an opportunity to cleanse and refresh itself. The experience is usually one of peace and well-being: people feel more in tune with the present and less caught up with memories of the past or fantasies about the future.

The deeper the relaxed state, the more potent its healing effect. Pain is another area where relaxation can help and people often find that they are able to experience relief from pain through practising relaxation. Some people, once they are relaxed, visualize or 'think' light pouring into the painful area. Others actually talk to their pain and see if they can find out what the pain is asking for. This method is described in *Getting Well Again* (see Recommended Reading).

## 1. Biofeedback

In the last twenty years the development of biofeedback training has done much to demonstrate the effects produced by changes in consciousness. Elmer and Alyce Green in the USA and Maxwell Cade in the UK have pioneered this field of research. Their work has revealed a great deal about the different kinds of awareness we are capable of experiencing.

Biofeedback uses a range of electronic instruments or meters which measure changes in electrical skin resistance (ESR) or skin temperature. These subtle changes are used to assess levels of relaxation or stress.

The ESR meter is perhaps the best known of these instruments and people are easily able to see how relaxed they are by checking the needle on the meter's scale. We can often think we are relaxed when in fact we are not, and biofeedback helps us to become aware of habitual or unconscious stress. Through relaxation, people are soon able to move the needle up or down at will. They learn to recognize the inner experience which corresponds with the relaxed state and so begin to retrain themselves, without effort.

Biofeedback is a valuable self-training technique which is used by many holistic cancer practitioners and centres.

## 2. Relaxation and visualization

There are lots of different relaxation and visualization processes which people use; these are often variations on a theme but each person may find that some variations work better for him or her than others. There are now many relaxation tapes on the market which may be suitable; with music, with guided imagery or visualization, or with straightforward progressive body relaxation.

It is perhaps useful to remember that the aim is to become a more relaxed person, rather than just the same tense person who does relaxation exercises. As with biofeedback, the techniques are tools to help you recognize the inner state and sensation which goes with being relaxed. Alternatively, they can also help you to recognize states of tension which previously went unnoticed.

It is often easier to start with someone else guiding you through the process, either in person or on tape. However, it is also easy to become too attached to that particular voice or source and to think you can't do it without them. If you can, try to learn to guide yourself mentally in relaxation. Eventually it is possible to become quite creative, making up your own variations to suit your needs at a paticular time.

Visualization or guided imagery is a powerful part of the relaxation process. It utilizes the relaxed state to create changes in perception, experience and even at a physiological level. The deeper the relaxation, the more potent the image.

People are often confused by the word visualization and think that they can't do it because they are not seeing clearly defined images. Some people do see inwardly in this way, but many will just have a vague sense of the image or even just the thought of it. If I were to ask you to close your eyes and imagine yourself getting up this morning, getting dressed and doing all the things you did right up to this moment, whatever you experience, that is visualization for you.

Visualization is perhaps another term for inner perception used in a conscious or deliberate way. Certain images seem to have particular effects. Clear water can feel refreshing and cleansing; sunlight, or soft golden light, can feel healing and soothing. Certain images are useful to create the idea of letting go — tying your fears and problems one by one to balloons and releasing them, for example.

The Simontons use a very specific set of images which aims to use the mind to destroy cancer cells and create a healthy growth. Patients are asked to get a mental image of their cancer cells and their immune system, or white blood cells. They then imagine the white blood cells attacking and destroying the cancer cells, getting rid of them as body waste and finally replacing the damage with normal healthy tissue. If the person is having radiotherapy or chemotherapy, then a positive image of that treatment is incorporated with the process.

Patients are encouraged to use this process twice a day. There are also certain guidelines which are seen as essential for the effectiveness of the technique. The cancer cells are best seen as weak and confused rather than as overpowering monsters. On the other hand, the white cells should be visualized as aggressive, powerful and numerous; an army of white sharks is one example of a suitable image. Treatment, such as radiotherapy, should be viewed as a powerful ally rather than a poisonous enemy. It is advisable to read *Getting Well Again* if you want to use this technique, because it is only a part of their whole programme.

Here is a suggested relaxation process which you might like to use. Twenty minutes is a good length of time. You can either sit or lie down, but beware of being so comfortable that you fall asleep. Make sure that your back is supported and that your legs and hands are uncrossed. It is a good idea to make sure that you are not disturbed, which can be bit of a shock if you are in a deeply relaxed state.

1. Bring your awareness into the present by listening to the sounds around you, both inside and outside the room. Let them come and go.
2. Bring your attention to the top of your head and imagine a wave of relaxation beginning to flow through that area of your body, melting away all tension. Allow that wave to flow downwards through each part of your body, jaw, neck, shoulders, etc. *Use your attention to systematically go through your body, from head to foot, until every part is relaxed.* If you like, you can use the idea of breathing relaxation in through the top of your head and breathing tension out through the bottoms of your feet.
3. When you have been through your whole body, take a couple of deep breaths. As you breathe out, allow yourself to feel more and more deeply relaxed.
4. You can either rest in this state for a while or go on to include steps 5, 6, and 7.
5. Imagine yourself in a beautiful, natural place; it may be a place you know or a completely imaginary place. Absorb the peace and beauty of this place. Really note the details of what is around you. What is the ground like beneath your feet? What does the air feel like against your skin in this place, etc.
6. Imagine that there are some balloons nearby and that one by

one you can tie each of your problems and fears to a balloon and watch it float away.
7   As you watch the last balloon float off, feel the golden warmth of the sun on your head and shoulders. Allow its golden radiance to warm and soothe your whole body, particularly the painful or diseased areas.
8   Gradually bring yourself back. Become aware of your body and the room you are in, and in your own time, open your eyes.

If you find your mind wandering don't worry, just gently bring your attention back to the process. Occasionally you may feel more tense or mentally agitated. This doesn't mean you can't do it, it is more likely to be the unconscious tension rising to the surface so try to stay with the process if you can.

## D. Mental healing

The holistic approach places much emphasis on psychological aspects of cancer. Negative attitudes and unhealthy psychological patterns are thought to play a crucial part in the onset of the disease. We experience our world through our perception and stress is governed by the individual's learned perception of what is threatening to them. The next chapter expands on this area and looks at some ways to let go of negative attitudes.

Whether or not you take view that cancer is caused by an unhealthy psyche, regular counselling or therapy can be an invaluable support in coping with emotional issues raised by the illness, as well as for discovering ways of using the situation creatively. It is also complementary to all other forms of treatment.

Being willing to take a good honest look at yourself and working toward a healthier approach and expression can take time, gentleness and a lot of courage. While it is something only you can do, it is a good idea to get the right support. There are more and more counsellors and psychotherapists who specialize in working with cancer patients, particularly those who use what is called the transpersonal approach. This newer and more holistic form of psychology includes the spiritual aspect of man, as well as the traditional areas of personality and the subconscious (see Useful Addresses).

## E.  Energy balancing

The idea that we are creatures of energy as well as form is an ancient one but one that is only recently becoming acceptable.

Kirlian photography shows patterns of energy emanating from living things. Even inanimate objects, such as minerals, show a field of energy. Analysis of the energy patterns emanating from hands show differences indicating health or imbalance.

Imbalances, or blockages in man's subtle energy system, relate directly to symptoms of an emotional, mental or physical nature. Therapies based on this principle, help to re-align the energy system so that a natural process of self-healing can take place.

## 1. *Acupuncture*

About four thousand years ago the Chinese discovered what they called *chi* energy, flowing around and through the body. They mapped out a fine system of energy pathways or meridians, running under the surface of the skin. These meridians relate to different organs and emotional or mental qualities within the person.

Although they are invisible to the eye, there are certain points on the meridians which are detectable to the acupuncturist. Ultra-fine needles are used to stimulate the acupuncture points and increase or balance the energy of the corresponding meridian.

In relation to cancer, acupuncture works holistically, strengthening patients and helping them to fight their own disease. If you are considering this form of complementary therapy, it is wise to make sure you consult an experienced practitioner and not somebody who merely uses the technique to get rid of symptoms. If in doubt, you can get in touch with one of the professional associations listed at the end of the book.

Acupuncture is also very helpful in relieving pain, without the disadvantage of side-effects. The Royal Marsden Cancer Hospital in Sutton, Surrey, now has a small acupuncture clinic for this purpose.

## 2. *Healing*

Healing is known by many names: spiritual healing, faith healing, laying-on-of-hands or hand healing. In all cases, the healer acts as a channel, receiving universal energy and transferring it through his or her hands to the person receiving treatment. The healer is able to locate energy blockages through the use of intuition and by feeling the quality of the person's energy or aura with his or her hands.

The art of healing is in many ways a highly subjective and individual one. For some it has religious associations and for others it is a purely natural phenomenon. Although it is possibly the oldest of all the therapies, it is perhaps one of the least recognized.

Many people associate healing with miracle cures and in some cases this does seem to have been so. However, in many more cases it may be a progressive therapy, where the whole person is effectively strengthened and their natural self-healing ability stimulated. This in itself can produce notable results. The client's willingness to recognize and heal any negative attitudes is also seen as essential for the therapy to be permanently effective.

Common responses to healing include deep relaxation, relief of pain, increase in vitality and an improved sense of well-being. Healers also tend to have a positive approach to death and do not usually view it as a finality. Helping a person through the process of dying can sometimes be an important part of healing work, enabling acceptance and easing pain.

Many cancer patients find regular healing an extremely helpful and nourishing addition to their treatment. It is even becoming more common for healers to be allowed into hospitals when requested to do so by a patient.

Some healers work through their local church, many of whom are beginning to reopen the tradition of a healing ministry. There are also associations, such as the National Federation of Spiritual Healers. Recently an Association of Therapeutic Healers was formed in response to the increasing number of younger practitioners who combine healing with other therapeutic techniques. Most healers have traditionally offered their services free of charge, but there is now a growing feeling that healing should be considered as a profession and take its place alongside the other branches of alternative medicine.

## F. Spiritual work

Within the course of daily life spirituality is about having a sense of purpose and meaning. Whatever the nature of our situation, no matter how impossible or hopeless it seems, somewhere there is a meaning and value which we can find and we can actively create. This does not negate the pain or difficulty but it is easier to bear. It means we can grow and learn from it in a way that is not diminished by our difficulty but is rather strengthened by it.

This applies to ourselves too. No matter how dark or unwanted some aspect of us may seem, if, like the frog prince, we can only allow and accept it, then it may transform before our eyes and reveal a value and worth that enriches us and expands our love and understanding.

Many people have found that cancer has provided that spiritual turning point of meaning. Through facing their own mortality they make a renewed choice to live, and discover a new sense of self and purpose in life. This sense is not dictated by events or length of survival but is rather fulfilled in each precious moment so full of opportunity for expression and love.

Spirituality is the discovery of an identity beyond our normal parameters of body and mind, a sense of self that is both intimately individual and universal at the same time; a sense of being loved and known beyond the barriers of our self-judgements and rejections; a sense of inner peace and wholeness, of connection to all of life everywhere, as part of a larger whole. This is the essence of holism, and one which embraces all cultures and religions, all people, and all forms of treatment. Each of us has our own pathway to that light within. We can use any thing, situation, relationship or moment as a tool to move us towards that place, including not knowing how.

If you are going to use any of the therapies mentioned, it is preferable if you can have the support of your doctor or GP. As I mentioned in Chapter 3 if you decide against having orthodox treatment your doctor may not be enthusiastic, but if you can at least have access to regular check-ups, your progress can be monitored. If you use vitamin supplements, it can also be a great help if your doctor is willing to prescribe them. If you have trouble finding a sympathetic GP, the British Holistic Medical Association may be able to help you.

As far as complementaries are concerned, choosing a practitioner is not always easy. Some therapies have professional associations, but in many cases, personal recommendation or word of mouth is the usual way. How well you relate to the practitioner is as important as the therapy itself and this varies from person to person. Always beware of anyone who says, 'I can cure you', or who promotes his or her method as 'the only way'. If he or she excludes and knocks other methods, they are less likely to support your own unique sense of well-being.

Each person will require a different combination of methods. If you are interested in a multi-level approach you may need to explore several possibilities before finding the right combination to suit you. A good practitioner will bear this in mind and may even have a referral system to provide for it. He or she should also be willing, as far as possible, to co-operate with any existing treatment you are having.

Most therapies are private and can be expensive over a period of time. Again, many good practitioners operate a sliding scale and are willing to negotiate if you are in difficulty. Healing is essentially an act of service and partnership. Lawrence Le Shan describes the health specialist as, 'a consultant, a guide "who knows the landscape", can make suggestions, offer alternatives, point out possibilities, help explore needs and blocks, but the process of designing a programme must be one in which the person for whom it is designed is a full partner.'

# 5.

# MENTAL ATTITUDE

People often talk about the importance of having a positive attitude, particularly in dealing with illnesses like cancer which seem to bring out feelings of helplessness and despair. Developing a positive attitude can make all the difference to a person's chances and speed of recovery. For some it can also be seen as the means of preventing further recurrence. There is increasing interest in the whole area of attitude, what it means and what effect it has on an individual's life and health. For some this has led to looking at how an individual's attitude can affect society as a whole.

There is a growing realization that we control our experience of our world through our perception. Our attitudes or mental points of view act like lenses, colouring what we see and we respond accordingly. Most of our attitudes stem from past decisions we made about specific incidents. They may have been appropriate at that time, but they then get programmed into our memory banks and become habitual. These habitual responses may have been conscious at first but after a while they become forgotten and unconscious.

When this happens we become somewhat restricted and mechanical in our response to situations. We can think that we see things as they really are, unaware that we have censored them to a large degree. We still act on the basis of the forgotten attitude. It's rather like seeing the world through a pair of spectacles which you forgot you put on! In this way the story of our past becomes the expectation of our future. We begin to see only what we expect to see, rather like the 'pickpocket who sees only pockets'. Like the vessel half filled with water, one person rejoices that it is half full and another grieves to see it already half empty.

Needless to say we have little trouble with our positive attitudes; it's the negative ones which make our lives difficult. Some people conclude on the basis of past events, that 'life is hard'. Even times of joy become reasons for cynicism as they await the expected betrayal or let down. As joy becomes more and more restricted, life becomes an ever increasing chain of evidence for hardship.

We can learn to reprogramme ourselves by becoming aware of the attitudes we hold and developing the ability to see things differently. By learning to change our attitudes we can alter our experience of our reality and increase our ability to respond to it.

Here is a simple exercise which you might like try, to test out this idea for yourself. You can do this on your own, writing down your responses or with a friend, taking turns to listen to each other.

1. Think of a situation or an aspect of your life which you consider to be an issue. Something which is a difficult problem for you. (I suggest that you start with a small to medium-sized problem and not the most major issue in your life. If you find the exercise useful you can then go on to apply it to other situations.)
2. Think about this issue as a really difficult problem, something which seems hard to resolve. Describe it to yourself or to your friend in these terms.
3. Close your eyes for a moment and notice what your experience was like as you described your problem in this way. How relaxed did you feel? Did you feel able to cope, or able to resolve the issue in any way?
4. Think again of the same issue. This time see it as a challenge, an opportunity to learn something of value for yourself. Again, describe your issue from this point of view.
5. Close your eyes once more and notice what your experience was like in relation to the issue. Did it change in any way? Did it alter the way you described the issue? Did you feel lighter about it? Were you able to see some purpose in having that issue? Did you feel more able to cope with it? Or, did you find it difficult to see it as an opportunity rather than a problem? Were you reluctant to let go of seeing it as a problem?

## A Time to Fight and A Time to Accept

There is an old saying that 'energy follows thought' which seems for me to sum up the implications of mental attitude. Our attitude can add energy to or lift energy from a particular way of thinking. 'Taking your mind off it', is a way of expressing what happens when we let go of a worry or fear.

I would like to explain briefly what I mean by the term letting go as I shall be using it throughout the book. People often think it means getting rid of something, when in fact it means releasing our emotional and mental attachment to the issue; and frequently involves a willingness to accept rather than resist. The situation may remain the same but we feel more detached and able to deal with it. We can then gain some peace of mind rather than increasing the burden of the fear and getting more and more caught up in it until it has a complete mental grip on us. One of the ways we can start to do this is by acknowledging the fear either to ourselves or by communicating it to someone so that we can begin to let it go. This need can be met by talking to a counsellor or friend. One of the main ways we hold onto and so increase the energy around a fear is by trying to deny its existence, pretending it isn't there. How often do you hear the reply to the question 'How are you?' as 'Oh, I'm fine', or 'I'm OK' when that clearly isn't the case?

I have also met people who continue to maintain the view that they are cancer patients long after their treatment is over. They have an almost obsessive interest in everything to do with cancer — memories of their operations, other cancer patients, etc., and they almost become professional cancer patients. Of course there is always a danger of recurrence but there comes a point when many decide that they might as well live their lives to the full without being controlled by the fear of getting it again. They may then begin to stop constantly thinking about what they are eating, worrying about every twinge or headache and they may at this point move away from support groups or even discussing cancer at all. Perhaps this is one of the reasons why we are not always aware of the many people who have recovered from cancer.

Sometimes people think that a positive attitude means 'You've got to fight it', in other words, keep going at all costs. While it is essential to have a fighting spirit, it may not always be the positive way to deal with a situation. If you think being positive *only* means fighting, then it can be very hard to let go — this is seen as 'giving in, giving up or failing'. Sometimes what is needed is in fact to let go, particularly when the body needs a rest or a chance to recover. Sometimes it simply means accepting the situation rather than resisting it. If this is what is called for, then it can be a powerful means of allowing a change to occur. One common example is the woman who, having finished a course of treatment, goes home and tries to carry on running the house, cooking, ironing, etc. Too much fighting spirit can produce more stress.

I have sometimes noticed that people can tend to deal with their illness in a way which only adds to their original stress pattern. In other words, their approach to treatment reflects and reinforces a negative attitude. One example of this might be someone who is habitually hard on themselves. This person then decides to fight the cancer by rejecting all help and going on a very extreme diet. They thus continue to purge and deny themselves any flexibility or pleasure.

Stress is a subject increasingly identified with cancer including the previously-mentioned theory that cancer is allowed to develop through stress-related suppression of the immune system. I have also talked about the work of Carl and Stephanie Simonton and their book *Getting Well Again*. Their self-help-orientated programme of relaxation, guided imagery and psychotherapy specifically uses mental attitude to regress cancer. Patients learn to identify and change habitual negative thought patterns as well as developing their will to recovery and health. They learn to adopt a positive attitude to themselves and to any medical treatment they are having. Patients are encouraged to set themselves goals for the future and to picture themselves achieving those goals in full health.

While goal-setting is a valuable tool in harnessing the will to live, sometimes there is a tendency to set goals too high. A step-by-step approach can be a valuable way of learning to realize goals. By starting with seemingly insignificant ones, you can begin to build a sense of confidence. Examples might be: 'Today I will notice three things I like about myself'; 'This week I will clean out the kitchen cupboards'; 'Tomorrow I will say "no" if that is my genuine feeling'. Taking one step at a time is a validating experience, whereas trying to leap too far, too soon, can reinforce feelings of failure.

## Relaxation and Play

Whether you agree with this approach or not, coping with cancer is definitely stressful. Learning to relax can at the very least help a person to cope with his or her illness. The various techniques mentioned in the last chapter are used by many cancer patients as they learn to go inward and let go of physical and mental tension. Practising relaxation in a group can increase the power of the experience. In the support group I was involved with, we ran weekly relaxation sessions where people knew they had a time set aside to be together and to relax.

One friend of mine took a relaxation tape into hospital with her when she had her mastectomy. She found it particularly helpful the night before and immediately after her operation. When my sister took a music relaxation tape into hospital recently, she found it had some unexpected uses. Her doctor was trying to re-attach her drip and was having great difficulty in finding a vein. After several painful attempts he, the nurses and my sister were in a high state of tension. She suddenly thought of the tape and suggested playing it. It worked; after listening to it, the atmosphere relaxed and they were able to accomplish their task.

Often just the day-to-day living, not knowing how it's all going to turn out, can be hard to cope with whether the situation goes on for a short time or over a period of years. Learning to live each day at a time without concern for a non-existent future is something that has value for us all. In a situation like cancer it can be enormously helpful. Again relaxation and meditation techniques help us to focus our awareness in the present moment. People often find that when they experience being totally in the present moment they have a sense of peace and well-being.

Sitting still and closing your eyes isn't the only way of relaxing. For some people, walking, swimming, dancing or other forms of exercise can be a good way; others might indulge in a luxurious bath, have a massage, or go to the hairdresser's. Anything that gives you pleasure can be a vital part of looking after yourself. Regular exercise is, of course, an important way to improve physical health and stamina.

Play, or 'feeding the child in us' as one friend of mine describes it, is something we increasingly neglect as we grow older. When we are ill, we can sometimes give ourselves even less time to play and it may be that illness is a time when we need it more than ever. How often have you been grateful for having a cold or flu because it gives you the permission to rest and do the things you like to do without feeling guilty about all your responsibilities?

Perhaps we all need to develop the priority of looking after the child aspect within us — allowing ourselves time to do really silly, light and 'funful' things. Children are playful, spontaneous, creative and loving and they like to laugh. If you don't give them love and attention they can become demanding, resentful, troublesome and extremely disruptive. Children are also known to 'get ill' to draw attention to their needs and to get out of doing things they don't want to do. This can become a lifetime pattern, which is perhaps food for thought. I find that if I don't give myself time to play I become restless and irritable. After a period of time I become tired and lacking in any inspiration. Alternatively when I go out and play, I can feel energized and regenerated.

Stephanie Simonton developed a simple exercise where you write a list of forty ways to play — twenty of which have to cost less than two pounds. You then make sure that you spend time each day doing some of the things on your list. Although I found it surprisingly hard to come up with forty things I like to do solely for pleasure, it occurred to me that playfulness is a quality I could bring to many of the things I do in my life — even the really purposeful ones.

The ability to say 'No' and to put yourself first is a part of this approach to life. It is frequently frowned upon as selfish, particularly in our culture. Many women have difficulty in saying 'no' and have traditionally been brought up to put others before themselves. This is a very noble attitude but I think we can become habitually over-generous and self-sacrificing when we don't really feel that way. It can be terrifying to say 'No' sometimes and take the risk that someone might be hurt or disapprove of your answer. It is important to have a respect and care for the gift of your own life. Being scared of putting myself first, and always doing what someone else wants regardless of my own needs, has drained me of strength and a sense of self-worth. It was probably one of the biggest causes of problems in my own marriage. At times it has filled me with resentment and guilt and has made the other person involved feel frustrated, guilty and resentful too, as they are trapped by my noble self-sacrifice.

It is a hard fact that you cannot live someone else's life for them; it means you take on their burden and sometimes deny them the opportunity of finding out for themselves. One friend of mine, Pam, who had cancer, experimented with this idea in what might seem a small way. She had a friend who was frequently miserable and who was always ringing up and wanting to come round. She knew that she could always lean on 'good old reliable Pam', who would always say 'yes' and would end up feeling fed-up, resentful and drained. One day Pam just said 'no' and was thrilled at the triumph of being able to choose for herself in this way.

One cancer patient said to me, 'I think it's a typical cancer patient's problem — being unable to say "no". You just end up whining and moaning and being resentful all the time. I'm learning to say "no" and it's great!'

## Judgement

This idea also includes what I call 'letting go of the *shoulds*'. I think we are often our own hardest taskmasters. We are always telling ourselves that we *should* finish tidying up before we sit down, or that we *ought* to go to the meeting or visit that relative when we'd much rather read a book. It's great to have the ability to do things you don't want to do but it can develop into an unconscious habit. Sadly it sometimes takes a crisis like cancer for us to appreciate the opportunity of enjoying our own lives.

Each time I find myself under pressure I look to see if there's an unnecessary 'should' or a 'must' hiding in there. Apart from anything, I find more and more that doing something just because I think I should rarely works out and is invariably unsatisfying. I don't mean that I only do things I feel like doing, but I try to give myself the opportunity to choose, instead of holding a big stick over my head and forcing myself to do something. Even if I do things because I think I should, at least I *know* that that's what I'm doing!

It is also easy to make positive thinking into a 'should'; in other words to tell yourself 'I *should* be positive' or 'I *mustn't* be negative'. That can cause stress too. One way of dealing with this might be to substitute the word 'can' and say, 'I *can* be positive', or 'I *can* stop being negative'. I find that this changes my own experience in a way that relieves me from obligation and gives me a sense of choice. It somehow contacts within me the ability to change, rather than imposing a standard which I feel unable to live up to.

This goes for feelings too. I think we often bracket feelings into positive or negative categories. Happiness, love, feeling good or feeling healthy are thought of as positive and anger, sadness, resentment or feeling ill are seen as negative. It is easy then to use the idea of positive thinking to reject those feelings and say 'I *shouldn't* feel angry or sad, I *must* feel happy and loving about my illness . . . I *should* forgive the doctors'. Sometimes however hard you try, you can't help feeling the way you do.

Perhaps it is possible to see feelings as just feelings — neither positive nor negative, but emotional responses that can be held with compassion and then released. 'I feel helpless and angry about my illness and now that I know I do and can express it, I can choose to let go of those feelings and begin to see a way to develop feelings of strength and well-being.'

Here is an exercise for letting go of negative thoughts and feelings. You can do this alone or with a friend. Doing this with a friend or in a group can make it more powerful.

## The Pool of Forgiveness

1. Close your eyes and begin to feel a sense of inner peace and stillness.
2. Take a few deep breaths. As you breathe out, imagine that you are breathing out all tensions and past thoughts. Breathe as deeply as you can.
3. As you breathe in, tell yourself that you are breathing in peace and stillness. Continue to breathe in peace and breathe out any negativity.
4. Imagine that in front of you is a pool of pure light, perhaps a shaft of sunlight. If you are with others, imagine the pool between you and link hands.
5. As you imagine the pool, start to think of some of the things you would like to let go. These may be things about yourself, or they may be about someone else.
6. Start to let go of these thoughts and feelings, releasing them into the pool. Breathe them out.
7. Say them out loud as you release each one, but as you let go, use the words '*I ACCEPT AND RELEASE . . .*'
   (For example: 'I accept and release my resentments about . . .' 'I accept and release my fear', 'I accept and release my anger towards my wife', 'I accept and release my thoughts', 'I accept and release my body', etc.).
   When there is more than one of you, take it in turns to say the phrases, letting go of each item one after another.
8. When you feel ready to move on, continue to let go aloud but this time use the words '*I FORGIVE . . .*'
   (e.g. 'I forgive myself for all the times I've hurt myself', 'I forgive myself for being afraid of dying', 'I forgive my husband for not loving me in the way I needed', 'I forgive myself for being overcritical', etc.)
9. Now open your eyes and in the same spirit of letting go, say '*I'M WILLING TO RECEIVE . . .*'
   (e.g. 'I'm willing to receive all the love and support I need',

'I'm willing to receive my mother as she is', I'm willing to receive peace of mind', etc.)

Perhaps a simple way of saying all this is to learn to let go of judging things so much. It is a universal human habit which often limits us and can add pressure to the things we have to deal with. For me, positive thinking is more to do with the quality of my experience — the way I deal with things rather than the things themselves. It is often as much to do with being kinder to myself when I don't live up to my own expectations as generating the will to achieve my goals. The art of positive thinking becomes one where there are no hard and fast rules but one with a number of useful tools which need to be applied creatively to each situation. The tools may change from moment to moment and from person to person — only you will know which is the right way.

One friend sent us a card with this verse on it shortly before she died:

> If I had my life to live over
> I would relax more.
> I wouldn't take so many things
> so seriously.
> I would take more chances.
> I would climb more mountains
> and swim more rivers . . .
>
> Next time
> I'd start barefooted
> earlier in the spring
> and stay that way
> later in the fall
>
> I wouldn't make such good grades
> unless I enjoyed working for them.
> I'd go to more dances
> I'd ride on more merry-go-rounds
> I'd pick more daisies.
>
> Frank Dickey

## Responsibility — A Sense of Choice
Responsibility is a word that is bandied around in the complementary treatment of cancer and it is a word that is

frequently misunderstood. *Responsibility doesn't mean blame or fault.*

We take on patterns of habit at an unconscious level and we are unable to do anything about that. In a single instant we experience so much that it is not possible for us to be conscious of it at all — sights, sounds, feelings and thoughts. We interpret our experience and select the most prominent or important aspects to be aware of. These selections happen as quickly as each instant follows one upon another and all the rest gets stored somewhere — in our unconscious. Regressive hypnosis demonstrates how the most intricate detail of a long forgotten moment can be made available to the consciousness.

Responsibility simply means ownership at a personal level — *'this is mine — I did it. Whether I was aware of it or not, it can be owned as a fact.'* What it then gives us is an opportunity to learn about ourselves from a place where we can experience a sense of choice and acceptance and ultimately the possibility of change.

I say 'possibility' because we may not always be able to change our circumstances, but by taking responsibility we can change the way we experience them. By doing this we can move from being a helpless victim to being an active participant, rather like shifting from the passenger seat to the driver's seat in a car. Responsibility also means 'the ability to respond' and it can enable us to deal a more effectively with the situation in which we find ourselves, even if it is a tough one like cancer.

Ultimately it is the ability to respond to our deepest truth — our own intuitive life force. It is a recognition of our own innate sense of rightness. The essence of life animates and creates all forms throughout the universe and, as such, carries that vastness of wisdom and power. There is no reason to suppose that we are an exception; each one of us carries a seed of that infinite wisdom. While it is common to all, it is uniquely expressed through each individual. By learning to trust ourselves, we begin to discover what life is seeking to express through us. By accepting responsibility we grasp the key to a treasure within and that has great power.

The first step usually involves coming to terms with our reality; being willing to accept our feelings and circumstances exactly as they are, without condition. Strangely enough this in itself can produce a powerful sense of freedom — a change in the way we experience something that takes the burden or significance of it away. Accepting something from the point of view of responsibility then begins to create this opportunity of choice, the opportunity that we can choose to experience our situation another way.

This was very much the basis of The Centre For Attitudinal Healing started by Dr Gerry Jampolsky in America. Dr Jampolsky works mainly with children who have life-threatening illnesses. He sees the children as his teachers and has written several books using their experiences as well as his own to illustrate his ideas. His two best known works are *Teach Only Love* and *Love is Letting Go of Fear*. Many centres have since sprung up throughout America and now in England, each developing in its own individual way. The main principles of the CAH are that:

1. The essence of our being is love
2. Health is defined as peace of mind
3. Healing is defined as letting go of fear

Using these principles, people learn to let go of fearful attitudes and develop their ability to see things another way.

The way my husband handled his chemotherapy was a good example of this approach. He was very resistant to the idea of chemotherapy. In his own self-treatment he was doing everything to rid his body of toxins by diet, visualization and mental attitude. He was confronted with the prospect of a treatment which he was told would save his life and if he didn't have it, he would die. He saw this treatment as being fed with more toxins.

He struggled with that dilemma which could be seen as 'If I have it I'll die and if I don't have it I'll die.' In the end he saw he could experience it another way and he chose to have the treatment and for it to work. He sat up all night with someone who was starting their course and watched their reactions, and saw that for himself he could choose to experience it differently. His response to the treatment was good and he had less intensive side-effects than many. He had very little nausea and was able to eat normally, putting on weight, which is the opposite to most people's experiences.

Another person who came to see us had just started radiotherapy. She was having some very intensive reactions of distress, diarrhoea and vomiting. She had had to agree to the treatment very quickly and was told that if she didn't have it she would die. She had been denied the opportunity of choosing the treatment and we talked about that. As it happened she had not been fully informed of the advised diet and had been eating all the wrong things. The hospital gave her a couple of days to recover before commencing treatment. In those few days she came to an experience of choosing and felt much calmer. Interestingly, she then decided to go on a raw food diet much of which was again contrary to the advised diet, but she never again experienced the same side-effects.

Some people have experienced that change in the cancer itself has stemmed their act of taking responsibility for themselves and their continuance of life. For each person the situation in which that happens or even the way it is expressed may be very different.

Dr Ann Woolley Hart had surgery for cancer some ten years ago and chose not to have radiotherapy. She describes her experience as that act of saying 'No', as if two halves of herself came together. She then went on to use homoeopathy and healing as part of her treatment. She took a tremendous risk in using methods about which she knew little but felt that the risk was worth taking. She has since become a champion of complementary methods such as homoeopathy and biofeedback for cancer patients, with a special emphasis on the need for personal responsibility.

My husband's expression of owning his cancer was, 'I created my cancer and if I created it then I can recreate it another way!'

My own view is that the act of choosing is as important as the form of treatment itself and I think many people can get sidetracked into thinking that it's the diet, or indeed the chemotherapy that's going to save them without really taking responsibility for themselves. It may not be to do with liking the form of treatment either (as in the case of Roger's chemotherapy). What I am talking about is choosing as a means of adding your will to the situation and that can be a powerful tool. As an expression of the will to live, the act of choosing can potentially release an enormous amount of life energy which can work for you. The various forms of treatment then become tools to harness that will and for each individual a different combination may be appropriate.

It is possible to think that taking responsibility is the answer to cancer and that doing so will guarantee a cure. Unfortunately, there is no such guarantee but a willingness to discover responsibility is an essential starting place. There are those who have not recovered in spite of adopting this stance, but perhaps they have found other benefits to be gained which have been of great value to them and have given meaning to their situation. Self-acceptance and quality of life bring a fulfilment which is not dependent upon circumstance or even physical outcome.

Many people are not willing to take responsiblity for their illness. It can sometimes take an enormous amount of courage to consider this and of course many people have recovered from cancer without even being aware of such a concept. However, I personally find it far easier to work with a person who is in some way willing to look at their part in the illness, and virtually impossible with someone who isn't.

Ultimately it is your illness, your treatment and your team of helpers. Recognizing responsibility is not necessarily an overnight process and may involve a long journey of continual searching, gaining insight and choosing over and again before deep change can occur. For some it may well be the experience of flipping almost overnight into another way of viewing their life followed by the lengthy process of integrating the implications of that experience.

In the words of one cancer survivor: 'Having cancer stopped me dead in my tracks, if you'll forgive the pun. It made me look at myself and ask myself, is this the person I really want to be? Do I really have to do all these things I think I should be doing? I was into over-achieving, I was career-orientated — I had such high expectations of myself. Since I've had cancer, I've become much more aware of my limitations. I think cancer makes you face up to the reality of your limitations.'

For some the whole experience of cancer has been an opportunity to transform their lives. I have often heard people say, 'I'm actually grateful for having had cancer.' They speak of having learned so much, that they now have a very different and much more satisfying experience of their lives that they hadn't previously realized was either lacking or available to them. Many have a more enriched inner life and creative expression and often wish to contribute what they have learned in some way. It is also common for people to let go of restrictive attitudes about time and the pressure to be always busy.

Obviously this is an opportunity that is intrinsic in any life crisis. From a holistic point of view, cancer would seem to have all the components of a need to transform one's life. At a spiritual level it is expressed in terms of a connection with the life force, of being a part of a greater whole and not isolated. There is the level of basic will to live, not only to survive but for this individuated life to continue. This is often translated into 'I have a right to live my own life and express it in my own way.' Tools such as the formation of goals are often used to encourage this — 'I'm going to be well enough to have a holiday this summer'. 'I'm going to stay alive because I want to see my daughter married next year.'

At a mental level it is expressed in terms of attitude toward yourself (self-worth) and who or what you identify yourself with (your job, your spouse or your children, etc.). Then at an emotional level this can be seen in terms of freeing repressed and denied emotional expression, particularly anger, resentment and grief, or simply aspects of yourself which you have never allowed yourself to develop.

Finally at a physical level there is the need to look after your body in terms of rest, good nourishment, exercise and environment. Many see the physical level of cancer as the last ditch stand of a message that Life is trying to get through to you, saying, 'Change is needed — urgently, now, for goodness sake, look, and if you don't look, that's it!'

It is very tempting for me to see cancer in this way and to judge people who have cancer on that basis. However, that would be a mistake too because a) I don't know all the answers to someone else's situation, and, b) I can see that possibly for some, cancer is a way of expressing something that has gone on for them. It may provide a sufficient release for the experience of losing a loved one, for example, or bring attention to loneliness and their need to be looked after. However, the continual habit of release through physical illness can be risky, especially if something like cancer becomes a form of expression.

For some people cancer is simply a way of dying — those who may have reached an age or time in their life when they are ready to go, rather than downing a bottle of pills, or even consciously realizing that that is what they want; get cancer as a natural and acceptable way to die.

I would like also to include a very small number of people I have encountered — three to be precise, who, I feel, had cancer for a slightly different reason. Two I met and one I never saw although I knew his wife. They all died and I believe they chose to have cancer as an opportunity of growing spiritually, the benefits of which went beyond Death. I don't mean they all went to heaven and were rewarded — but they saw it as a major part of their spiritual development through and beyond this physical life. One of the three expressed this point of view directly, explaining that he had to go through the process of dying of cancer for what he described as his 'group spirit' to evolve. Another had expressed his certainty of reincarnation and implied that his illness was a major growing point in his own continuum. The third person never spoke of this: she had chronic leukaemia for twelve years. This is in no way evidence but just my own opinion about her and the way she accepted what was happening to her; the phenomenal amount of learning she did about every aspect of the subject of cancer, and also the incredible courage with which she persisted throughout her illness.

Whatever the interpretation or the level of opportunity that people perceive — whether it is the courage to finish a relationship which no longer works, to let go of a job that is killing you, to evolve spiritually or simply to get well and look after yourself better — the opportunity is there. Whether it is held as a reason for cancer occurring or simply as a sensible way of coping with it, it can be a creative and enriching way of drawing benefit from the whole experience.

# 6.

# RELATIVES AND FRIENDS — THE SUPPORTERS' EXPERIENCE

> Love is more than simply being open to experiencing the anguish of another person's suffering. It is the willingness to live with the helpless, knowing that we can do nothing to save the other from his pain.
>
> — Sheldon Kopp

Perhaps the most obvious thing to say about relatives and friends, is that they have an experience of cancer too. However, their needs often get pushed aside in order to give priority to the patient. There is still a lack of information and support for relatives of cancer patients. One response to this need is a book by Stephanie Simonton, called *The Healing Family* (Bantam Books, 1984).

It may seem a strange thing to say, but it is sometimes easier to cope with a situation if it is you who are in it. If you simply have to watch someone else, particularly someone you love very much go through a crisis, it can seem harder because there is nothing you can do and you are not always sure what kind of resources they will have to cope with it all. If you are diagnosed with cancer, people are often busy fussing around you, pouring on love and support. That's as it should be; but if you are told that your wife or father has cancer, then you sometimes have to handle that news alone, unless you make a conscious effort to seek support.

Shock, the fear of losing a loved one, not knowing what to say or do, yet wanting to appear strong, loving, cheerful and supportive, are among the multitude of responses which can flash through your mind in those early days. Perhaps the person who is ill has always been your staunch support, the one you always relied upon when you were down and didn't know what to do.

Now they need you — but who can you go to?

It is easy to push those feelings aside by telling yourself that you shouldn't need help or support because after all, you're all right — you're healthy. You may even feel guilty that they have cancer and you don't. I know I felt dreadfully guilty about asking for help. I really felt that I didn't have the right, because I didn't have cancer. Thank goodness I had some decent friends who were good enough to keep prodding me and telling me it was OK for me to be looked after too. So remember that you do have the right and that you may have more need than you sometimes realize. After all, the patient is probably aware that you are hanging on to unspoken tensions which they are unable to take on. It will ease their mind if they know you are being taken care of.

Things can also become quite intense if you become the target for the patient's pent-up reactions. As the one closest to them they will feel more able to express their feelings of distress to you. You then have to deal with their response as well as your own. This can be particularly so with men who often have a tendency to bring all their feelings to the woman in their life, rather than seeking outside support.

It can seem easier to cope with it all if you plunge yourself into *doing* things. Your life becomes a mad whirl of to-ing and fro-ing from the hospital, fetching and carrying, coping domestically, giving out family bulletins, seeking information from books, friends, acquaintances and doctors. Relatives can sometimes become even more avid information-seekers than patients. Your helpfulness can take over their experience if you are not careful and you can end up by swamping them with advice and suggestions which they may not really want, or which they would rather find out for themselves.

This approach can be a way of coping, but it can also be a trap. In order to avoid that terrible feeling of helplessness, the temptation is to do it all for them, to emotionally take on the illness, stress and strain yourself in the hope that it might make things better. Of course it doesn't, although it is a very natural human reaction. It is easy to underestimate the depth of our need to avoid the experience of helplessness. It wasn't until a year after Roger's recovery that I became aware of this. I was shocked when I realized how much I had tried to take on his experience in order to avoid my own feeling of helplessness. I realized how hard it can be to allow someone else to suffer, to remain compassionate and to just let it be.

Trying to do everything yourself may also be a way of proving how much you love the patient. The only problem here is that he or she may end up more worried about your ability to cope. In my own case perhaps the hardest thing of all for me to accept was the plain fact that there was nothing I could *do* to make it better, to take it away. It wasn't my fault that my husband or sister had cancer. And yet, perversely, there was something I could do. I could accept that this was their experience and their responsibility and I could trust them to pull through. That giving of trust can in itself be of positive support. 'I trust you to do what's best for you and I'll be here by your side. You let me know what you need and I'll be here to remind you of the love we share and to provide something familiar and warm in the midst of all this uncertainty.'

It's easy to forget how much just being around, just being there, means to a person who is going through the loneliness of a major illness. Perhaps in the end, it is the most important thing of all, that *you make a difference simply by being yourself.*

Another common tendency is to think that you haven't done enough, 'there must be something else I could do, if only I'd done more, perhaps if I'd done such and such then this wouldn't have happened.' You can torture yourself with these kind of thoughts but in the end you have to come to terms with the fact that you can only do your best and that that is enough.

Protecting the patient, deciding what to tell them and what not to tell, is an issue which many relatives have to deal with. Surrounding the patient with love, positivity and cheerfulness is important. However, while it is good not to burden them unnecessarily with every single problem, denying any bad news or pretending everything's going fine when it isn't can sometimes be diminishing. It can effectively take away the patient's ability to handle their own situation.

It is a difficult point and one which can only be settled individually. Perhaps one of the key questions to ask yourself is, '*Am I doing this for them, or am I really doing this to make me feel better, because I can't cope and I'm scared?*' It comes down to trust again. 'Can I trust my loved one to handle it, no matter how bad things are, or do I deny them the opportunity of ever finding out whether they are capable or not?'

Perhaps some people are better off not knowing how ill they are, or that they are going to die. I don't know the answer to that one. As I said in Chapter 3, I have met people who were absolutely convinced that in their case, they were right not to tell.

What I do know is that it must be a terrible burden to live with someone and not be able to share things openly, no matter how bad. In my own case, I had to handle a particularly difficult situation, perhaps the hardest I've ever had to face. As I've already mentioned, Roger and I were in the process of splitting up when his cancer was diagnosed. In a sense, cancer forced us to stay together at a time when we needed to have some space and distance from each other. Because of his violence towards me I was terrified and desperate to get away from him, but he was critically ill and he needed my support. I resented being with him but I also felt dreadfully guilty that I didn't experience the love and support I wanted to feel. At the same time I was terrified that if I did leave him he would die and I'd never be able to forgive myself. As a result of this impossible conflict, I was secretly wishing he'd die because it seemed the only way out of my dilemma.

Admitting this to myself was very hard, but hiding it was even worse. In the end I realized that, given the way I felt, perhaps leaving him was the most supportive thing I could do, and I was only able to do this by going to talk to someone who I knew would listen to my feelings without judging me. When I finally plucked up the courage to tell Roger, I was surprised and relieved to find how well he took it. He already knew how I felt and however upset he was, he just wanted to get well and to have the right atmosphere and support around him to do that.

In sharing the experience with him, I stopped treating him as a cancer victim and he became a person again, an adult who had the right to know what was going on and with the ability to share things. I had to trust him to live or die for himself and I left not knowing but with a sense that what I had done was right.

As it turned out he did get well. My leaving gave him the opportunity to choose whether or not he wanted to recover and to find within himself the capacity to deal with his own illness.

This was an unusually difficult situation, but it does happen. Those guilty thoughts about wishing your partner would die because it seems like the only way out, or the nasty nagging ones about hanging on for the benefits of the insurance policy, do come into nice people's minds and they won't go away. It's a relief if they can be shared. I don't necessarily mean with your partner, but at least with someone who won't hold judgement over you. If you feel you could benefit from counselling, enquire through your hospital social worker or one of the listed support group networks.

The focus is always on the patient and if you don't have someone to talk to, you can even end up resenting that too at times. Friends and visitors call and ask, 'How is he, is he OK?' but often not asking you how you are and again you may feel guilty about asking for attention. Meanwhile there you are, silently in the background, being noble and trying to push away your needs. Perhaps you wish you could forget it all and get away from cancer for a while.

In the cancer support group I was involved with, relatives rarely came forward. They seemed to melt into the background, giving space to the patients' needs. In most cases, people are fine and happy with the way they are coping, but if they're not, how do they deal with it?

It can be lonely living with a cancer patient at times. If the person is physically low, they may just want to rest and may not feel like talking. As I have mentioned, radiotherapy and chemotherapy often make people feel very tired and even depressed. This can also be quite hard to live with. It can take months to recover from a course of treatment or an operation and you can feel housebound and isolated while the person is recuperating. The treatment itself is rarely an overnight affair and may be spread over several weeks. If cancer recurs, then the whole process is repeated, sometimes over a number of years.

When you're not looking after the patient at home, then you are travelling back and forth to the hospital. This in itself can be demanding, especially if the hospital is a long way from home. Much time is spent hanging around, anxiously waiting for the patient to tell you what the doctors have told them. Developing the ability to take each day as it comes is just as important for you as it is for the patient. The picture changes all the time and you have to be able to adapt to the periods when the patient's energy is low and their morale is hard to sustain — then your encouragement becomes all the most important.

If it is your partner who has cancer, it is easy to feel shut out of their experience. However close you are to them and however much you want to share the situation, there remains that factual difference in your experience and you are always one step away. When several patients get together, they can seem rather like members of an exclusive club at times, swopping hospital experiences etc., with you on the outside.

If someone is very sick, you might be afraid to leave the house even for a short period and yet shopping has to be done, food has to be prepared. People do not always realize that they can apply for a home help if necessary. One woman I knew, looked after her husband for four years before she discovered she was entitled to have one. She hadn't had a day off in all that time.

There is, in fact, a self-help organization called the Carers National Association which was specifically set up to help those whose lives are under stress through having to care for someone. Volunteers can help out for short periods, so relatives can have a break or even a short holiday while they know things are being taken care of.

Time off is essential and if you are drained or stressed then you are less able to be supportive in any case. It can be easy for cancer to dominate your existence and yet you are often the patient's link with normal life. If you can take time to enjoy yourself and do things which give you pleasure, you are then able to share that enjoyment with your loved one and provide some lightness and relief. It is common for relatives to think that they mustn't enjoy themselves because someone they love is ill.

It may also be good for the patient to have some time away from you too. You can get on top of each other after a while and a change of company can be good for both of you. It is all too easy to get stuck in a rather unhealthy guilt syndrome, where the relative ties themselves inextricably to the patient and finds it impossible to leave them, even for a second. Even if you go out for half an hour, mentally you are still at home, worrying that something has happened and feeling guilty because you're not there.

If things don't go well and you are facing the prospect of bereavement, it can obviously be a most difficult time for any relative. Your job is to give support and yet in the end it is you who are going to be left behind needing someone to support you. The feelings of anger and grief well up inside and the temptation may be to hang on to them until it is all over. Sometimes it is possible, with help, to release some of those feelings now. They are part of a natural process of adjustment. If you let go, rather than bottling them up, it may leave you freer to be with your loved one and share that time together.

If you are able to communicate openly with each other, it can be a great help; you can face and accept things together. If, however, you have decided that it would ease things for the patient by not telling them, then you may have to hold on to your feelings and keep going. Again, receiving counselling, going to a support group, having someone to talk to, can all be of great help at this time. The suggestions made in Chapter 3 about writing things down, or drawing the way you feel, can also be useful as are any of the points in the chapter on mental attitude.

Sometimes you may find yourself going through a kind of mental rehearsal of what it would be like to be without that person. It is easy to feel guilty about having these kind of thoughts, but they are part of nature's way of helping us to adjust.

One of the difficulties is that doctors aren't always able to predict how long things will take. Human beings are often far more enduring that we imagine — three months can stretch to six, or even eighteen. In the end it still comes as a shock, all the 'doing' and 'keeping going' suddenly stops and you are left with yourself.

Bereavement counselling is becoming quite a specialized field these days and there are several organizations as well as individual counsellors who deal specifically with helping people through the process of bereavement. The best known of these is CRUSE which is a network of local branches, each operating in its own way. Services range from support groups, to one-to-one counselling and home visits, and all volunteer counsellors are specially trained. Compassionate Friends is a similar organization which offers support to newly-bereaved parents.

I am aware that parents of children with cancer must have particular problems and needs apart from those already mentioned. Having a child with cancer can be an extremely challenging experience to accept. There seems to be little information available to cover this area and although I have no relevant experience and am unable to ease that situation I would like to acknowledge the need. I would also like to add that hospitals are very accommodating and understanding when it comes to the emotional needs of parents and children in this situation. I often wish that kind of open support were available to adults in the same predicament.

I have found one book called *Children With Cancer (A Handbook for Families and Helpers)* by Merren Parker and David Mauger (Cassell Ltd, 1979). This book was written in New Zealand and is quite comprehensive when it comes to the emotional aspects of dealing with this situation.

Gerry Jampolsky, as I have already mentioned on page 81, has done a great deal of work with children with cancer. His books are available through some bookshops and also through the London Centre for Attitudinal Healing. The Centre also has some tapes of Dr Jampolsky talking about his experiences. I have seen two American TV programmes featuring Gerry and some of the parents and children who come to the Centre in California. Perhaps the overwhelming thing for me was to realize that children are people who are able to relate to what is happening to them with dignity and maturity. They are often able to exhibit more acceptance and openness than adults, even when it comes to their own death. The Centre's programme encourages the children to support each other and runs pen-pal schemes. They even have a special arrangement with the telephone company, so that children can call each other across the States, free of charge.

There is a holistic centre for children with cancer in the UK, based in Orpington, Kent, and I have listed the contact address at the back.

Being close to a person with a major illness can have its positive side. Many people find it brings a greater closeness to a relationship. For me it has been an incredible opportunity to contribute and to serve the ones I love. It stretched my resources to the full, but it also strengthened them in a way that would not otherwise have been possible. I have a much deeper understanding of myself, of others and the predicaments people sometimes have to face. Strangely enough, it has also increased my sense of trust in people and in life, regardless of the circumstances.

# 7.

# LETTING GO

**Death as a Process of Change**
As I sit here during the aftermath of Christmas celebrations, trying to write this chapter, I am aware of a sense of ambivalence toward the time of year. To me, Christmas is very much a contrasting experience of life and death. One year's cycle draws to an end, 'only sixteen shopping days to Christmas' and the pressure is on to get everything done before the doors close on 24 December. It is supposed to be a festival of birth, yet I discover in myself some weird fantasy which heralds the twenty-fifth as my death date. After then I imagine my life will be over and January looms ahead like a vast, cold, black void. I doubt my ability to survive it all and panic mounts.

December always seems to be the shortest month of the year, one minute it's begun and the next, it's Christmas. Each day becomes more and more intense, the call to express abundance and celebration somehow brings forth an experience of its opposite. I become painfully aware of all that is wrong in my life; loneliness and poverty, inadequacy and anxiety.

This year, as I sank into my usual panic and depression, for the first time I began to see it as an opportunity to observe rather than *be* those negative aspects of myself. I saw my darker side which seems bent on destroying any chance I have. This is the side of me which wants to die. Everyone of us has this side to our personality and when it emerges we become identified with it, thinking of ourselves in terms of failure, fear, loneliness and poverty. I asked myself the question, 'Who is it who has these feelings?' At that moment I transcended this view and saw these feelings as facets of my personality but not as the essential me, and I suddenly felt like celebrating. A sense of joy which you could call the Christmas spirit was born in my heart. Christmas is a celebration of birth after all, but one which is transcendent. I found in myself a deep appreciation for death and the opportunity for cleansing and growth which it represents. For me birth and death are inseparable; in order for something new to be born, something has to die. It is interesting that in Christian terms, the birth of the Light of the World happens when the earthly cycle is in the midst of dying. Equally, Christ's death is celebrated in Spring, when nature is in the midst of giving birth.

I sense that the undercurrent of December death is felt by many. It is a fact that more people die around this time of year than at any other, yet we choose to ignore or defy it all by boldly stepping out, buying and giving, eating and drinking to excess. It doesn't matter about tomorrow, after all it's Christmas! It all strikes me as rather like the person who have been told they've got only six months to live and who reacts by going on a cruise and trying to cram in all those things they never did before.

Perhaps it is easy to be philosophical or detached about death when not immediately faced with its prospect, yet the truth is that we are all terminal and could go at any time. Somehow we choose to ignore that fact and do a marvellous job of convincing ourselves that there will be a tomorrow or a ten year's time. Most of us shore ourselves up against experiencing the possibility of death and then when it happens we have a hard time coming to terms with it all.

It is within the realm of our experience that we have to deal with death. I believe that we constantly have a taste of that experience and for me, it is always linked with the process of change. The prospect of change has often looked to me like death; a time when I would cease to be. Once, when I faced up to the fact that I needed to give up a twelve year career as an actress, I experienced an acute sense of shock, loss and disorientation. I felt as if the person I had been was gone for ever, that I had no future, and I was terrified. As I allowed myself to move with that deep process of letting go, I noticed that each day passed and each day someone got up. As the tremors ceased and the period of grief and mourning passed, I realized that something had remained. It had been the idea I had of myself and my life which had passed away. Somehow it had become such a firmly engrained view of myself that I could not see any other possibility and prising it loose was painful.

During those months of disorientation, I just accepted each day as it came and experienced a strange lightness and sense of peace. I no longer knew how to identify myself and yet I felt an intense awareness of the beauty of the blossom on the trees and the stillness in the air.

Looking back, I can see how fitting it was to let go of that identity. It had more than run its course and it had to go in order for something new to emerge. It seems amazing to me how painful it can be to let go of something so unreal — a set of ideas. Although I can give no concrete evidence, I believe that physical death is no different, a loss of identity or form which reveals a continuing essence or consciousness.

As a healer, I have had a small amount of experience of working with dying people. The sense I have got has been very much of taking part in a delicate process of preparation, but a preparation for transition rather than ending. I have had a sense of building a connection with something immense and powerful yet full of love and acceptance. I have at times felt more like a midwife than anything else. It seems to me that healing can be of great help in the dying process, making it easier and less painful.

The concept of death as a link in the continuum of change is familiar to Eastern minds, but to Western culture it is an alien one. In fact alienation accurately describes the state of relationship we in the West have evolved toward death. We have placed so much emphasis on prolonging physical survival, on 'saving lives', and have developed remarkable skills and equipment to this purpose. We have achieved many miracles of which we can be proud, yet within this context death has become the equivalent of failure and is seen as the grand invalidation of all our schemes.

We seek to hide this indiscretion by denying it all, by whisking away the deceased before anyone sees them, by disposing of the departed cosmetically and cleanly. We have become what is described as a death-denying society.

This seems strange in contrast to the utter obsession we have with violent death when it comes to the media and entertainment. The media tends to focus on the unordinary, the dramatic. I remember once attending an educational seminar on world hunger. It was pointed out that we mostly associate starvation with famine and yet that factor only represents one tenth of the total number of deaths caused by hunger. The reason for this is because famine is an unusual event and therefore counts as news. It was then I realized how much I am exposed, by the media, to the drama of extraordinary, so much so that I find myself accepting it as representing ordinary reality. In terms of death,

I now find myself automatically associating it with war and violence. No wonder we are frightened of death and want to push it away. Anyway it's safe on a television screen while we sit immune in our chairs, able to switch off if it all becomes too unbearable.

However, death isn't always like that and by pushing it away we no longer become able to include it as a natural part of our life, or to see it as an experience to be valued.

We push away the dying too, we hide them in geriatric wards and other institutions. People rarely die at home any more, they go to hospital instead. Often, when someone is dying, doctors carefully avoid the word and say with regret, 'There's nothing more we can do'. That just about sums it up. What a terrible indictment that we think there is nothing creative we can offer the dying, that they have no needs or indeed that they have nothing of value to offer us. Again it boils down to the over-emphasis on quantity at the expense of quality. In simple terms of human friendship and caring there is plenty that can be offered. Just because a person's physical machinery is packing up doesn't mean to say that they themselves don't have mental, emotional and spiritual needs.

### How Can We Let Go?

Fortunately we have begun to redress this balance with much creative work now being done to improve our understanding of death and the quality of care given to those who are terminally ill.

There are currently several excellent books on the topic of death, particularly by American authors, some of whom write with humour as well as perception. Ram Dass, in his book *Grist for the Mill* (Wildwood House Ltd, 1978) talks about death in a chapter called 'Dying, an Opportunity for Awakening'. He shares his views and experiences on the topic, including a surprisingly humorous yet compassionate description of his mother's funeral. His co-author, Stephen Levine, has become noted for his own work on the subject. His books *Who Dies?* and *Meetings on the Edge* (Anchor Doubleday, 1982) are particularly recommended.

One of the names which springs most readily to mind as a contributor within this field, is that of Dr Elisabeth Kübler Ross. A Swiss-born psychiatrist, living in America, she has devoted her life to learning about and caring for the dying. She has been a major pioneer in helping to change attitudes. Her first book earned her the nickname 'The death and dying lady' (*On Death and*

*Dying*, Tavistock Press, 1977). Elisabeth Kübler Ross is a compassionate woman whose wartime experiences, helping concentration camp survivors, gave her a deep understanding of life and death issues. After qualifying she began conducting hospital interviews with the terminally ill. She developed these into seminars where medical staff sat behind two-way mirrors while volunteer patients talked about their experience to her and a colleague. There was much hostility towards her work at first but it gradually became recognized as a major break through. Those who attended the seminars felt very moved and learned a great deal from the people they listened to. Most important of all, the patients themselves, overwhelmingly appreciated the opportunity to share and relate to their experience, as well as being able to offer something of value.

Dr Kübler Ross has described the natural response to dying in terms of five emotional stages. These stages do not necessarily occur in sequence nor are they always completed, but they provide us with a valuable guideline for recognizing the person's needs. They enable patient and supporter alike to work with the process rather than against it, to a person's needs rather than imposing anything on them.

She regards death as a unique opportunity for growth and sees the patients as her teachers. Great emphasis is also laid upon the value of expressing and releasing some of the intense emotions people have in relation to their death.

**Stage One** — is denial ('*not me!*'). Disbelief can be seen in a positive light as it may provide a person with the time to orientate themselves until they feel ready to face the news. Some people choose to stay in this state right until the end and in this case their choice should be respected.

**Stage Two** — is anger and rage (as an expression of '*why me?*'). These feelings can often become channelled toward family and medical staff. It is vital that they be recognized for what they really are and that the person is encouraged to express them fully. Dr Kübler Ross includes physical expression, such as cushion hitting, etc.

**Stage Three** — is called bargaining ('*yes me — but . . . !*'). This is when a person attempts to postpone the fateful day by pretence or pleading for it to be put off awhile, 'just till after my daughter's wedding', etc.

**Stage Four** — is depression ('*yes me*'). This represents recognition of fact and is a deep experience of loss or grief. It can be seen as a necessary phase of mourning for the dying person and that cheering up or jollying along is inappropriate and inhibitive to the process at this point.

**Stage Five** — is acceptance when a person has let go of all the resistance and has finally come to terms with the experience.

It is interesting to note how similar these responses are to those experienced by people when first diagnosed with cancer. My own feeling is that they are common to all situations of change which involve the experience of loss and that they manifest more or less intensely, according to the significance of that which we are losing. Whatever the circumstances of change, whether it be physical death, loss of a job, divorce, or even loss of a breast through surgery, the natural healing process of letting go seems to be the same. First comes recognition, followed by grief and mourning and then finally acceptance.

Another important aspect is letting go in terms of close relationships. This usually involves communicating any unfinished business, the thoughts and feelings lurking around from the past, still unexpressed. This applies to both the person who is dying and their family and friends. They may be feelings of past resentment and frustration, they may also be love and appreciation. The simple words, 'I love you' usually lie underneath all the bad stuff but until that has been expressed a genuine experience of love can continue to elude us.

This incompletion can cause problems for those who are left behind. How many of us have felt this kind of regret and frustration in relation to a deceased loved one, 'If only I'd told him how much I loved him'? You might find the 'Pool of Forgiveness' exercise in Chapter Five a useful one for dealing with 'Unfinished Business'. *Getting Well Again* (see Recommended Reading) also includes useful material for handling resentment as well as a guided imagery sequence for dealing with feelings about death.

We often give resentments far more significance than they really have. We preserve them in guilt and then bottle them up inside where they lie, gathering poison which damages our relationships and peace of mind. I find it helpful to remember that resentments don't have to be fair, nor do you have to make the other person responsible for them. They can be communicated simply as an expression of your own feelings which need to be heard.

Completing relationships on a practical level is also a very important part of letting go. If it is possible to discuss financial matters such as wills and insurance, or even funeral arrangements, it can all help to add to the peace of mind of the dying person. They are then able to feel satisfied that everything is being taken care of as they would wish.

Active participation in the funeral arrangements by relatives is becoming recognized as an effective way of helping to ease the grieving process. In Kübler Ross's book *Death the Final Stage of Growth* (Prentice Hall Inc., 1975), an undertaker writes of his own realization of this when his father died. He has since begun to encourage and support his clients in this way. In Britain, Jane Warman, who ran a bereavement counselling service in London, encouraged people to arrange what she calls 'do-it-yourself funerals'. It was through the experience of creating and arranging her mother's funeral along with family and friends that she appreciated the value of participation

Finally, the willingness to let go of the relationship itself needs to be faced. If members of a family are unwilling to let go, then it can make it harder for a person to die. Sometimes relatives and even doctors will try to persuade a person to have treatment they may no longer want. Patients may have come to terms with the fact that they are going to die but often give in because they don't want to hurt their loved ones.

Only recently I met an eighty-year-old woman whose consultant was trying to persuade her to have a highly complex and unpleasant operation which would have prolonged her life rather than eased her death. Her comment was, 'If you can guarantee that I won't come through the operation, I'll have it'. This might be seen as sufficient indication of her needs, but for a while she agonized over giving in for the sake of her family.

It is important to remember here that letting go means giving up the attachment to the relationship and not getting rid of it altogether. Being willing is the keynote and it can, in a strange way, leave you much freer to be together. Suddenly there are no more conditions, only the present moment to be shared, and there is much peace and joy in that.

When a relationship has a sense of completion, when there are no longer any hidden issues between us, we can have a much fuller experience of each other. There is an intense experience of love, a sense of peace and an increased awareness of being in the present. There is nowhere to get to, nothing to achieve, just an experience of being here now. It need no longer be an issue of how long we survive but of the qualities of life we can express now.

## Terminal Care

Perhaps death is the greatest opportunity we have to meet the challenge of what it means to be human. The dying process might then be translated into an experience of intensive living and this view is shared by those who specialize in terminal care.

The rapid expansion of the hospice movement in recent years has helped to fill the gap in the health service. The emphasis is on caring and responding to the whole person's needs. Hospices (meaning 'home of rest') originated as resting places for pilgrims and the religious aspect has taken on a broader spiritual view within the new movement.

The hospice aims to provide a loving, informal and peaceful environment where people have an opportunity to be looked after, while living as fully as possible, until they die. It is a place where they can die with dignity and according to their individual wishes, rather than at the convenience of others.

It also provides much-needed relief and support for families whilst fully encouraging their participation. A common misconception about hospices is that once you go in, you never come out, but facilities range from home care, day care and short-stay to permanent-stay. Patients may be based at home but come for short periods in order to give families a rest, or to stabilize pain.

Families can come and go as they please and are often encouraged to help look after the patient. This is seen as a useful aid in adjusting to and easing the bereavement process. Bereavement counselling and follow-up support is usually available to families for several months after a patient has died.

Pain relief is seen as a first priority but, unlike the approach of many hospitals, the aim is to remove the physical discomfort without clouding the patient's mind. Hospices have become skilled in developing the right balance of drug dosages which enable the patients to retain as much clarity as they need in order to cope.

Listening, physical contact and friendship are all seen as intrinsic parts of the service which are offered unconditionally, as and when the patient or family needs them.

Hospice teams include medical and nursing staff, social workers, physiotherapists, chaplains and many lay volunteers. All staff are carefully selected and trained. Their own adjustment to death, ability to cope, and emotional needs are seen to be as important as the care they offer. Provision is usually made for staff support.

In this country, hospices have mainly developed as separate entities but are complementary to the hospital service. The accepted forerunner of the modern hospice movement is St. Christopher's Hospice in Sydenham, S.E. London, founded in 1967 and pioneered by the redoubtable Dr Cicely Saunders. St. Christopher's has become a world centre and inspiration for the development of and research into terminal care. There are now over one hundred hospices in this country.

The Cancer Relief Macmillan Fund has developed the Macmillan Service to cater for the needs of the terminally ill. A small number of Macmillan units have so far been built within hospital complexes and basically provide short-stay facilities. The emphasis is again on individual care, pain control and family participation. Cancer Relief also fund the training of Macmillan Nurses who provide terminal home care (also referred to as continuing care). The Marie Curie Foundation is another charity which arranges this type of service.

Home hospicing is a very recent development in this country and there is a growing awareness that many prefer to spend their last days at home. Some hospices have developed teams who can provide the kind of domiciliary care which will allow a person to stay at home. The United States has mainly adopted this approach to hospicing with the emphasis on enabling the person to return home wherever possible.

Some hospitals have begun to recognize the need for care when cure is no longer available and there are a few which have special units providing a similar service to hospices. The inclusion of this type of facility within the hospital system must be seen as a positive step towards providing a more complete health care service. It is surely preferable to retain links with the doctors and staff who are already looking after the patient. Perhaps the spirit of love and teamship offered to the terminally ill could be just as well applied to any hospital patient or health professional.

Canada has been particularly successful in developing this type of facility, largely due to the work of Dr Mount, an oncologist at the Royal Victoria Hospital, Montreal. He is a great believer in the importance of including the hospice ideal within the hospital service.

Terminal diagnosis and how much a patient should be told is still a question to be considered. The answer, I feel, must and should depend upon the patient, with the doctor being willing to provide as much information as he or she wishes. Again, there are instances where families have decided that it is better for the patient not to know and the state of denial is maintained to the end. This may be total or part denial, where there is unspoken knowledge and verbal pretence. The doctor has to provide a cue for the patient by asking them, in some way, how much they wish to know. In the end, surely it is a person's right and need to have the opportunity of coming to terms with their own death.

Another question is that of how much the doctors really know and when should we finally give up hope of recovery. When doctors give forecasts on the amount of time left to a person, they are frequently accurate, but there are also many instances where they have been wrong. There are even cases where doctors have given time scales and yet patients have recovered. In the end we have to admit that nothing is certain.

## A Matter of Identity

> Death is that which allows life to be born.
> The old form drops away . . . so!
> It is but a pause in the breath of life;
> Love death, love life for they are one.
>
> Death is merely the loss of an idea,
> How strange that a mere idea can be so painful!

We have so little trust in the unknown, even when what we know is intensely uncomfortable or destructive to us. And so we fear death, the greatest unknown of all. We spend our lives trying to pretend it doesn't exist. Within this pretence we are able to ignore and hide so many of the things which we find uncomfortable. But they do not go away and in the face of the mystery of death, all the hidden unwanted things well up to the surface, as witnessed in the process described by Elisabeth Kübler Ross. It seems a pity that we so often wait until the event of physical death to confront the unknown. Death doesn't only concern the dying. Perhaps if we were more willing to live with the unknown, we wouldn't hang on so long. We wouldn't store up so much of the fear of which we would dearly like to rid ourselves. The unknown could be seen more as that which allows possibility to be born, a place to be embraced as the source of our being instead of its annihilation. In this context death becomes more to do with the rigidity which results from clinging on to unwanted things rather than letting go of them.

For me, a key to it all seems to lie in the words identification and attachment. To the degree we see ourselves as identified with that which we need to let go of, we feel pain and loss. If, for example, who I think I am becomes my work, then when I lose my job, I think I will lose my existence; I will die. If I see myself merely as a physical body and personality, then I think that who I am will die along with these.

These ideas are central to many religious philosophies, particularly Buddhism which preaches the attitude of non-attachment. Who I am becomes the mystery which is formless and cannot therefore be described, only experienced: pure consciousness or awareness that creates form and imbues it with the quality of life.

This may all seem like very abstract philosophizing but for me it all has a very real day-to-day effect on the way I experience my life.

Western civilization has become adept at exploring and understanding the world of form. We are also a highly individualistic society, upholding the sanctity and importance of the individual identity. The more holistic or communal identity, such as seen in Eastern countries, terrifies us. We fear loss of individual identity and power and see only grey uniformity. We tend to associate this kind of identification with countries where the communal priority has been imposed, rather than naturally expressing the people's perception of themselves.

Whilst individuality is important it also increases a sense of separation. Separation serves the purpose of enabling us to distinguish ourselves from our environment and indeed, each other. It enables me to discern the difference between my experience and yours, so that I don't have to react a certain way just because you do. This is valuable in creating healthy personal relationships.

If separateness becomes our *only* view of existence, we are bound to have more difficulty in letting go of anything which represents our individual identity. If, on the other hand, we see ourselves as part of a larger organism, as unique and individual *expressions* of the continuum of life itself, then individual survival takes on a very different meaning. Who we are becomes more akin to the kind of power which keeps the Universe going, the stars twinkling in their billions and the sun warming planet Earth as it turns and turns.

For much of my life I saw it as being up to me alone to keep my world going, to keep the whole show on the road, and that was a struggle and a failure. More recently I noticed that something far larger than individual me makes it all work and that I must be part of it. When who I am becomes identified with the very force of life, then how can I die?

As George Bernard Shaw said:

> This is the true joy in life, the being used for a purpose recognized by yourself as a mighty one; the being a force of nature instead of a feverish little clod of ailments and grievances complaining that the world will not devote itself to making you happy. I am of the opinion that my life belongs to the whole community, and as long as I live it is my privilege to do for it whatever I can.
>
> I want to be thoroughly used up when I die, for the harder I work the more I live. I rejoice in life for its own sake. Life is no 'brief candle' to me. It is a sort of splendid torch which I have got hold of for the moment, and I want to make it burn as brightly as possible before handing it on to future generations.

# 8.

# 'WHERE DO I FIT INTO ALL THIS?'

On Monday I gave up smoking. I chanted 'Today's the day I give up smoking!' twenty-five times and that was that. I haven't bought any cigarettes since. It's been dreadful — stripped of my pretence, my prop — I'm left alone with frightened, needy me. On Wednesday I stood on the pavement outside the house for a full ten minutes, poised between will-power and addiction. I told myself I could buy a packet and come down slowly; 'I'll smoke one a day,' I said to myself. No sooner had I said that when the voice in my head said 'Well maybe two a day' and I thought 'O-oh' as the voice of my sanity exposed the voice of self-delusion.

As the untrapped energy surges around me reaching out to grab, I start to snack again — munching anything to feed the void. The unblocked energy explodes and last night I was up till four, not knowing what to do with myself and reading a passionate feminist biography until my eyes burned with fatigue.

The hungry child in me shows no discrimination. Choice died nameless years ago as I learned the habit of feeding myself Death and now I don't even know how to begin to enjoy nourishing me with Life. The few times, the odd peak experiences when the terror has abated and tranquillity has reigned, I have been blown away by the feeling of simply breathing in Life. There is something out there after all, something that fills me, caresses and cares for me. Ninety-nine point nine per cent of the time, my senses are dulled by fear and only the acrid smoke of death is able to block the pain. There's never enough, I must have more, and another firestick burns into my chest. That familiar feeling of mucus in my throat and thoracic tightness has brought strange comfort over the years as it became more prominent than the real pain inside.

On the other hand, each ragged sore intake of breath only adds to the mound of guilt that I am slowly 'doing myself in', then releases itself in a long sigh of anger and self-pity.

Now I'm left with the symptoms, no longer distracted by the contents of a packet of JPS. Even Herbalife can't protect me from the pangs of hunger that search around for respite; I acknowledge my doubts that I can survive without food for my nameless addiction. For three years now, I have seriously battled with giving up smoking — cutting down from thirty to four a day, then up to twenty, down to ten and in between, weeks, even months without any at all.

Roger and I tried to parent each other out of it, making and breaking agreements with each other, catching each other out with tenacious lies and justifying our failures. Roger used to send me out on the street like a ponce, persuading me to whore for cigarettes from passers-by. My need drove my guilt and I'd make up stories: 'Excuse me, I wonder if you could possibly let me have a cigarette, only I'm baby-sitting and I can't leave the house to go and buy any?' Responses would vary from silent refusal to unwanted generosity as sympathetic addicts pressed three or four 'life savers' into my embarrassed hands. Then the shop across the road started to sell single cigarettes, in response to economic decline. For us it was a day of rejoicing, now we could legitimately ration our habit with self-prescribed doses.

One day I came home, trying to forget the near empty packet of ten in my handbag. Roger said 'How many have you had today?' 'Two,' I replied, with thin conviction. 'How many?' he repeated with absolute certainty. He wasn't heavy, just persistent, laughing all the while at the ridiculousness of the situation. He even said 'Look, I promise I won't get angry, just tell me the truth; I know you're lying.'

My pride kept a grip on me as my mouth clung to my lie. Inside I watched myself with amazement and laughed at the farce of it all. Two climbed down to four as he persisted with the question 'How many?'

Then the plot took a new twist as he changed the question to 'Did you buy some today?' 'No,' I pleaded. 'Let me see your bag.' 'Look I haven't bought any.' 'Come on, let me see.' More giggles, as we both wondered how far this thing was going to go. 'All right, I bought some . . . but I threw them away so I wouldn't have any more.' That one went down well . . . for a bit, then the persistence resumed until finally Roger found the packet with two left and the curtain came down.

We laughed at it all but inside there was the sadness and knowledge that I was no different from any other addict, alcoholic, heroin or otherwise. Let's face it, death wish is death wish, whatever the poison.

Sometimes Roger would question me and I would think it was to catch me out, but it would turn out that he only wanted a fag himself.

When he had cancer, that was the real spur. Although it wasn't lung cancer, it was a reminder that he should respect the lucky break he'd had and learn to look after himself. I was guilty by proxy and supporting him was my motive.

Even though we have long since parted, we still battle on. His puritan 'cancer survivor' act can't hold out against the closet addict and organic raw food temporarily gives way to chips and nicotine sticks once more, and so it goes on.

Four weeks ago I ventured down to the basement of myself and pulled out the aspect I call 'Poor me'. She is terrified of the world and yet now she's here, in living colour, what do I do with her? Another aspect of me I discovered down there, is called 'Pigso'. He is her companion and lives on burdens. He doesn't know how to exist without them.

Yesterday I was aware of taking something with me to Betty's, just because I feel naked without a burden in my hand. I'm always carrying a handbag and then buying things, little, useless things, that I have to clutch in brown paper bags, until my right arm aches and finally I make it inside the front door.

I'm never without something to carry. When I was with Roger, it required a conscious effort and felt really strange to go out without anything. I'd ask him, 'Have you got the key? Have you got some money?' No more excuses left and I'd have to leave my security handbag behind. Uncertain and vulnerable, I'd step out of the front door. Never truly alone, not even for a few seconds. After all, even though I didn't have my handbag, I had Roger.

All my life, I wonder whether I've ever really stepped outside the door alone and trusted to life to breathe me and feed me. Yes, by comparison to most people I live a life of cliff-jumping — a freefall sort of existence. But do I really?

I must get to the bottom of this. My healing gift nudges me toward the possibility of feeding myself life instead of death. Perhaps I can slowly learn to be whole, healthy, beautiful, slim, peaceful and, God forbid, happy. After all I've had enough of the alternative and I'm sick of putting up with my fear. Today's the day I heal my addiction, today's the day I heal my addiction, today's the day I . . . etc.

On Wednesday night I dreamed I went to Pluto. For the first time I have a strong sense of remembering. It was a deep experience — Pluto is the planet of transformation and self-awareness after all. Through the darkness comes the dawn. I remember being given a crystal ball, I gather we all placed them in our hearts since we couldn't bring back the physical manifestation. I have a feeling I will though — I mean that I will get a real crystal ball from somebody. In the meantime, it's in my heart where it really matters as I look into the depths of myself to find the light. Pluto figures large in my birth chart and since the last psychosynthesis workshop, I've taken to wearing black again, symbolizing my first journey down into the basement of myself. 'Poor me' was covered in soot in a blackened cellar, when I found her. Now she's progressed to wearing blue occasionally and I discovered she really has blonde hair (just like my sister, what a coincidence!?).

I used to wear black to hide my figure, to make me look slimmer. These reasons still linger, but I also know I'm wearing black right now as a symbol of my commitment to know myself — not to hide, but to bring the full me out here into the sunlight for healing.

Now my sister has cancer. Three or four weeks ago I wasn't surprised but surprisingly shocked with the news. Diana, my big sister/mother, the family focus, everybody's organizer. Diana, the moon goddess, having trapped herself in the unwanted role of Ceres the earthmother, finally rebelled.

After the first wave of grief and self-pity, I push the feelings away; it's all too close. I despair of ever being cancer-free, it's always surrounding me. An ex-husband, the hungry needs of a cancer support group, and now, as I sit writing my commissioned advice and comfort book for cancer patients, the threat of death comes through my door once more.

I was actually in the middle of writing Chapter 2 about treatment and struggling to find the right balance between frank information and reassurance. It's depressing; there are so many side-effects. The treatments seem almost as daunting as the illness, except that your chances of recovery from treatment are higher than from cancer. It's the only option most people have and I try to stay objective. It is important that people have a positive attitude toward their illness and treatment. People need to be informed but they also need strength and encouragement.

I feel I manage to maintain the balance with my own integrity, but it is hard and somewhat depressing. After all it's easy for me, I've never had cancer. I begin to see how tempting it is to fall into the conspiracy of protection that most medicals do, and I feel compassion.

Then comes the awful news; a rash of emotions well up, past fears. I automatically slip back into overstrain; the crisis pitch I managed to sustain for all those months, three years ago; God knows how? It's not the same, I keep telling myself. I'm no longer struggling to cope with Roger's irrational explosions of terrifying rage which left me like a paralysed rabbit striving to stop the breach in the dyke against a tidal wave. I no longer have to wrestle with the anguish of wanting to give love and support while fighting against the desire to run.

This is different, this is my sister now. This is a happier scene — a family that rallies round and supports. All the love and caring come spontaneously. Any feelings that get locked away are normal fears of the worst and stiff upper lips thrust spouses into action instead.

Diana herself is plunged into almost immediate transformation — I am amazed at the speed with which she addressed the issue. At first all calm, it hasn't really sunk in yet: 'I'm going to be all right you know'. She takes to the Simonton book and the realization that this is all about her as a person and her need to grow and change, not just a death-threatening physical illness. She realizes that her cancer is a symptom — a warning.

A week later it all breaks open. She calls me to her hospital bed and is drugged to the eyeballs to cope with her first chemotherapy. She is in despair, her life has fallen apart. Motherhood, her biggest investment, gone with one fell swoop of the surgeon's knife. What does the future hold for her now? That's the real fear, 'What will I do in my fifties, my womb gone and my looks fading fast?' She says she is more afraid of the future than of cancer.

Then in her delirium she drifts from future to past and in floods of tears and anger she bewails her lost talents. I've never heard her talk this way. She has artistic gifts, gifts for dancing, singing, writing, and all she ever got out of them was years of typing other people's letters, tickets to Covent Garden and a ten-year struggle to bear her own child.

Although I share her grief, in my heart I'm so glad. I am astounded as I watch my forty-eight-year-old sister open up her feelings to me for the first time — the birth of the person behind the role. For the first time in my life I am able to offer her something. I understand the pain and confusion of growing and at last she understands me. We bridge the gap of communication that has frustrated me all these years. I know she'll be OK.

She says, 'I'm not afraid of the cancer, it was a warning and now I've got the message, I don't need it any more, it's served its purpose!' I feel incredibly moved to hear her say this.

I realize that she and I are like yin and yang, we've contrived to develop opposite sides of ourselves at the cost of the other half. This year seems to be a rebalancing for both of us. I recover from my own crisis, having come out of a fruitful but terrifying marriage that nearly cost me my will to be myself. I broke myself trying to fit into what I thought I wanted — but the part of me which really wanted nourishing hardly got fed at all. The process of my leaving was very much like one of looking at the 'cancer' in me. It was an issue of self-denial, and of the stress that was being created. This year I learn to put myself together and gingerly to come out of my dream, fantasy world where it's safe to masturbate on my own talents but stop at material success. Inner sensitivity at the expense of worldly achievement.

For my sister, it's the opposite: domestic and financial bliss, but inner starvation. I cheer for us both; Life refuses to give up on us and we have the sense to follow it through.

I am moved with admiration for both her and Roger, whose exceptional courage is an example to all. Perhaps it was too much of an example because Diana admitted to me one day: 'You know, ever since Roger got cancer I feel I've been gearing myself up to it. Almost as if I gave myself the thought, this might be good for me too.'

I feel strongly that cancer is often a self-induced symptom of the personality's need to heal or make itself whole. Having watched two people go through such a plainly needed transformation it seems impossible for me to ignore, quite apart from all the countless others who report a similar experience. Yes, for me it is an unconscious expression of the need to change from a way that no longer works. The challenge is to take responsibility and acknowledge the need rather than simply struggle with the symptoms. The body is a machine which houses the person and it is the person who makes the difference in that house, not just the bricks.

Of course this doesn't mean that the cancer doesn't matter;

the physical has to be looked after too. No matter how much change a person is willing to undertake, the risk is always there. I'll never forget Rob Thomas who did everything in his power to turn around his life and address his needs, yet he lasted only a year after his melanoma was diagnosed. However, I do not believe he died in vain. He learned a great deal about himself in that year and inspired many others by the way he handled his illness with such openness and sense of responsibility.

If it wasn't for Rob Thomas, Roger wouldn't have known where to start when he was diagnosed only months later. He wouldn't have known about Bristol, the diet or the whole self-help approach. He wouldn't have known that suffering rebels are also made of pioneer stuff. And, if it wasn't for Roger, Diana would not have made such rapid sense of spiritual change and conquering the incurable, and so on it goes.

Here's to all the people who are willing to wake up to the reality of themselves, to those who are willing to lose all they seem to have in order to find something far greater that they really had all the time! To all who find the courage it takes to be responsible (and it does take plenty) I salute you!

Life will answer if you are willing, finally, to trust in her. After all she bore us and she beckons to each and every one. As I learn to let go and respond, I find that she does know what's best for me in the end. I thought I had to struggle for survival in a threatening world and my reality lovingly shaped itself to my command. Now I'm learning to take things easier and let life do the work. To do otherwise is to beat my head against the wall. I'm learning to ride the horse in the direction it's going, as they say, and it's great! Each day is one of adventure and mystery, of gifts and miracles; I simply have to learn to see more clearly. If I should die next week, or next year, I know my life will not have been wasted. It fulfils itself moment by moment, in the quality of its expression.

In the words of Hamlet:

> There's a special providence in the fall of a sparrow.
> If it be now, 'tis not to come: if it be not to come,
> it will be now; if it be not now, yet it will come:
> the readiness is all.
>
> *Hamlet V ii (232)*

# 9.

# PATIENTS AND DOCTORS

As previously mentioned in Chapter 3, the patient/doctor relationship is often far from easy. The traditional roles of authority and passive victim which we are conditioned to play, are slow to change. On this score, doctors have become the target for much criticism from the general public and have been accused of lack of care and consideration for patients as individuals. However, it is easy to overlook the fact that they are just as bound by their role as we are by ours.

In the light of this current climate of mistrust, I felt very strongly that I wanted to include a joint contribution from both doctor and patient. I was fortunate enough to be able to arrange such a discussion between my sister and her consultant, Dr R. H. Phillips, a consultant radiotherapist and physician in oncology. The following dialogue is extracted from a conversation which took place between the three of us shortly after my sister received a diagnosis that the cancer had reached her liver.

I cannot thank them both enough for their willingness to cover this difficult subject so openly and so fully. It is a tribute not only to them as individuals, but to the value that such a positive relationship can bring to the field of health care. I hope it may also bring a strong ray of hope in redressing the balance.

### Extracts of a Conversation Between a Doctor, a Patient and the Author

Dr      What was your reaction when you first heard the diagnosis?
Diana   I suppose deep down I'd known all along.
Dr      Was it a relief when it was confirmed?
Diana   Yes. Funnily enough, if we skip several months, to the

| | |
|---|---|
| | last diagnosis I had. That was also something I was fearing. I was very deeply depressed during the whole of that time, but when it was confirmed it was like a load had been taken off my mind. |
| Rachael | Dr Phillips, how often do you think that patients already know inside? |
| Dr | I think that the vast majority of patients know, even those who outwardly give the impression that they do not. |
| Rachael | Of course, in Diana's situation, you didn't come into the picture until after she was diagnosed, so you weren't the person to break the news to her. |
| Dr | Yes, that's right. Was it broken to you as 'this is cancer'? |
| Diana | Well, we knew the results of the test had come through and my husband told me.<br><br>I think one of the interesting things was when I had a talk with the surgeon, the night before the operation. It was as if he was almost willing me to ask certain questions and waiting for me to given an indication of how much I wanted to know. |
| Rachael | Is that true in your experience? |
| Dr | Most patients come to me after the diagnosis has been made, so they may have been told that they have cancer. There is then a whole variety of possible reactions. A certain number adjust to the knowledge of the disease very quickly and are very keen to proceed with further explanation of the treatment options. Some put the information to the back of their minds and will deny that anyone has spoken to them about it, because this is the way that some people cope, by keeping things privately to themselves. Others may not have been told the diagnosis, and there are still quite a large number of patients who will have worked it out for themselves, but no one has actually sat down and explained it to them directly. A small number will have no idea that the illness may be malignant and may not ask any relevant questions at all.<br><br>It is my firm belief that the patient needs to know what is going on, because the implication of that diagnosis and the subsequent treatment is such that I feel it is their right to know. I, personally, find it very much easier to help patients and to treat them fairly and, hopefully, with success if they do have the basic know- |

ledge about the illness. Then we can talk together about the problems when things are going well and also, with trust and confidence, when they are not going so well.

Diana  How much do you take your cue from the patient as to how deeply you are prepared to go into the diagnosis and its implications? I think I have certainly found it easy to establish a very frank relationship with you, but with certain other doctors I have had to work harder. I have been very conscious of the fact that it was as much my responsibility as the doctor's to establish what sort of relationship we were going to have. Because I happen to be a person who likes to know exactly what's going on I have been at pains to make that quite clear.

Dr  We certainly do take cues from the patient. With someone like yourself, it was very easy, because what I believe and what you want actually coincide — so there is no problem. We can go ahead and discuss things in full with all the implications. In many situations it is extremely difficult to predict what is going to happen, so we can only discuss matters in general terms. Without being evasive, and trying to be absolutely honest, you cannot be terribly specific. Now there are other patients who will say 'Look, you're the expert, you carry on and I'll take your advice' — just as I do with my accountant, when I say, 'you sort my money out and I'll pay the bill' but that's my big hang-up. There are some people who wish to establish this type of dependent relationship, and that's fair enough as well. It doesn't mean that we would not wish to discuss the various options very fully with them, and I still think it is very important to discuss the treatment and what the likely side-effects are. Once again, there is a certain amount of tailoring to individual needs and personalities, as there is in personal relationships at any level. There are some people to whom we relate very easily in social contacts and others with whom we have to work a lot harder.

Rachael  So what you're saying is that being a doctor is no different from being a human in any other situation.

Dr  That's right — you're a human being needing to establish an interpersonal relationship with a patient, but with a very difficult barrier between the two. I say barrier very specifically because it is a hurdle for me as much as it is for the patient. I think it is very important that people don't run away with the idea that it's easy for a doctor to spend his life telling people they have cancer, to be continually delivering bad news in a highly emotive area.

Rachael   Do you think this is why some doctors are very distant?

Dr   Yes I do, absolutely. I don't think we should criticize individuals who find it difficult. I think there is an intrinsic fear of the disease for many of us and to a certain extent we don't know how we would handle the problem if it happened to us personally.

Rachael   There's an area in my own work which I have had to address again and again at deeper and deeper levels. As much as I know it intellectually, there's always a part of me which thinks that I can make somebody else better and I don't believe that is true. However, if I can let go of the need to make somebody else better, for me to cure them, then perhaps I can create a much more helpful environment in which they can find a way to heal themselves.

Dr   You mean a more realistic scenario than holding onto the cure when, if this is not achieved, you feel a complete failure.

Rachael   Yes.

Dr   I think this is a very potent concern for many doctors and other health care professionals.

Rachael   How did you feel, say last week, because you had to give my sister a very poor diagnosis?

Dr   Awful — it was not at all easy. To a large extent, it does make it much more difficult to manage this sort of situation if you have established a close personal relationship with a large degree of empathy. I saw the scans and the report, and we talked about them, and I was as disappointed as I knew you were going to be. Oh yes, I wasn't looking forward to meeting you, but I knew that from the basis of our relationship that I would have to tell you what was going on. There was no question that I would not tell you, but the disappointment that I felt was very real, as it always is.

Diana   Well, I think it must be so, because from that point of view you've chosen a very difficult field to work in. Fairly early on, I started talking to you about vitamin

| | |
|---|---|
| | supplements and various things that I wanted to try myself . . . |
| Dr | Yes, indeed, did you find that very difficult to bring up? Were you worried about how I'd react? |
| Diana | I wasn't worried about you by then because I'd got to know you. I was somewhat worried when it got to the first point where I had to say, 'Right, I've got very politely to give you the sack and I'm going off to Bristol to try different things.' I must say I was very warmed by your reaction and the reaction of the gynaecologist as well, but I had felt all along, that if I just sat back and let someone do things to me that it was not a very satisfactory situation for me to be in. My morale was better when I could do something for myself. Twice I have made this decision, as we know, and each time I have felt much lighter, as if I didn't have so heavy a burden to carry, although in a way I was giving myself a bigger burden because I was taking this responsibility on myself. How do you feel about this aspect? |
| Dr | I think it's of fundamental importance that people feel they are taking an active part in the decisions regarding their treatment and, indeed, in the treatments themselves. Once you start to take a different diet and you have to be prepared to change your lifestyle, then you are positively contributing yourself in an active way. For many people this is important and for their families as well. I think this is where complementary forms of treatment are very valuable in that they emphasize the whole concept of self-help and involvement. I don't know what the figures are for the results of these various treatments, and I suspect that it may be very difficult to glean the exact scientific statistics. Some of the more conventional treatments that we are involved in are beginning to be designed to involve patients' families much more in the management of their own malignancies. For example, chemotherapy and home infusional techniques, which we're very keen on, can make a tremendous difference to our patients. Instead of coming into hospital each time for an intravenous drip, a tube is inserted into the vein which will stay there long-term and the patient may pick up the drugs for preparation and administration in the home situation |

| | |
|---|---|
| | — this is a very positive step towards involvement in the treatment. |
| Rachael | My view is that taking charge of yourself in some way, that the act of taking responsibility and expressing it by choice, is crucial. How important do you think that is? |
| Dr | Yes, I agree that this is a very important point. |
| Rachael | It seems to me that conventional style treatment and the way that the whole relationship is generally set up, can tend to reinforce a sense of helplessness. |
| Diana | I think it's very easy to sit back and be a victim, I mean you're a victim of the disease and you're a victim of the treatment. You're in this helpless situation and the doctor comes along and says, 'Right, I propose to give such and such a treatment', and you're grateful because you're very frightened and you accept it. But, after that initial acceptance, you start to think about things. Just as you say, 'OK, the accountant will advise me, but in the end I pay the bill,' so the patient is paying the bill in that sense. It seems to me that it's up to the patient to say, 'Look I accept your professional advice but there's a dimension that I have to contribute.' If the doctor is an understanding person then it is easy. I suspect that with certain doctors this is not very easy, but I don't think that any patient should grumble about being treated as a number, as I heard someone say recently. If they feel like that, I think it's up to them to assert themselves. I know it's difficult when you're feeling very ill, but there are moments when you're not feeling ill and you can think about it. |
| Dr | I think it's very sad to hear that particular statement. I am sure there are patients under our care who feel they have been treated this way and I very much regret it. There is a question of time; you need a lot of time to do this properly and there are many pressures which exist. This can be a terrific problem as you have to cover such a vast amount of work that you can't necessarily provide for every individual patient what one feels is needed in terms of psychological, as well as physical, support. I think you have to qualify your earlier statement about wanting to take control of your own destiny, which I agree with entirely, by considering the individual characteristics of each patient. Some are not |

capable of, or willing to do this, and they want to be completely taken over with every bit of responsibility falling on the doctor. To treat the patient as merely a number, though, is unforgivable and each individual should be given full and sympathetic consideration as a human being who happens to have cancer. It is something that we in the medical profession have to be very careful about, because there is a great deal of routine work and these are diseases we see every day of the week. However, for each patient it is a unique experience and it is very important that we keep this at the front of our minds. We are dealing with unique individual human beings and not just with disease processes.

Diana  Do you consciously pass this attitude on to the staff who work with you?

Dr  I do try as much as I can to do this.

Rachael  Going back to the last meeting you had a couple of weeks ago, which was obviously very difficult for both of you, I wonder if you would be willing to say a little more about what was going on inside?

Diana  ... What was interesting was that in all our time together, there is one question I have never asked you and I think you know which question that is: 'How long do I have?' I felt all along that you were bound to say it could be such and such, but in a sense I didn't feel it was your responsibility to tell me, because I felt that ultimately it was up to me.

Dr  You have actually answered the question as I would have answered it. In just the same way that you cannot be absolutely sure of the level of response in an individual patient, similarly you really have no idea how the disease is going to behave and, therefore, what the time span will be.

Rachael  And yet a lot of time doctors do make those kind of pronouncements.

Dr  Well, maybe they do, but I generally don't. In fact, the times when I have made such decisions, for example, should relatives come from abroad, I have almost invariably been wrong. I have said, 'I think you ought to come now' and six months later the patient is still around.

| | |
|---|---|
| Diana | We've talked about the relationship between doctor and patient, what about the relationship between the doctor and the relatives? |
| Dr | With our relationship, the dialogue has been between the two of us. This doesn't apply to every patient or family by any means. There are some families who make a conscious decision that their relative will not be told. They say, 'You mustn't tell him, it would kill him.' Now this does happen and it is a reflection, not of how the patient will react to this knowledge, but of the problems the families feel they will encounter in coming to terms with open and frank discussion of the situation. |
| Rachael | Do you ever feel it is valid not to tell people? |
| Dr | Very occasionally. I have to respect the views of the immediate relatives, but I do say that if the patient asks me a direct question I will have to answer truthfully. However much I respect their view, if it comes to it I will not be able to lie. I also feel that it is an insult to the intelligence of the patient asking me this direct question to withhold the truth and if this is done it merely adds to the frustration, isolation and anxiety which the patient may feel. From my point of view, the most difficult relationships are very often with the families, because the patients and I are directly involved. When it comes to the families, they may feel very distant, frustrated and completely impotent and unable to help. |
| Rachael | I think that coming to terms with the fact that there isn't anything you can do is a very basic issue. I think as humans we will do anything to avoid feeling helpless and when watching somebody else suffer we will do anything to try to make it better and to try to make it better for ourselves. That must be true for doctors as well as relatives. Until you've really come to terms with that impotency, you're always putting pressure on them or doing something to cover it up. That's what I was talking about earlier.<br><br>It has taken me four years to really learn that. I had to learn it with Roger and now I'm having to learn it with Diana, but I feel I've reached a place now where I truly don't have an investment in her result. Ultimately there is something very powerful you can do just by being there with them and not having any needs of |

| | |
|---|---|
| | them. It gives the patients more room to choose for themselves. |
| Diana | This is true, one is very conscious of the sorrow that those close must be feeling. Even though you are the central issue as the person who's doing all the suffering, at the same time you feel protective towards your loved ones. For instance, I have been absolutely frank with everyone right up until last week and then I made a conscious decision not to tell my parents. They live closely with us and have been a great help. No doubt life would have been much more difficult both practically and emotionally if they had not been around. But it's easier for me at this stage not to have them looking at me and knowing what's going on in their minds. Also Jeffrey didn't want them to know because he finds their concern difficult and, if I'm honest, part of my decision was to protect him from their concern and make life easier for him. |
| Rachael | How often do you encounter the situation where the patient knows and the family doesn't? |
| Dr | It is quite common and sometimes the doctor is caught in the middle of a very aggressive situation. Relatives may be very upset if you are not doing what they consider to be the correct thing, and this is sometimes a very difficult problem to come to terms with. When you are really trying hard to help someone, and the response is anger and criticism from the family members who are, in fact, taking out all their guilt and pressures, all their fears and anxieties on you. They can't take it out on the patient because of the protective element and so they find the nearest person, who happens to be the doctor. |
| Rachael | Do you see this as part of your job? |
| Dr | Yes, I think it's a safety valve for some people. |
| Diana | You asked me earlier on how I felt at the initial diagnosis. It was amazing how so many emotions just came welling up to the surface over the period of weeks, feelings from the past that I wasn't terribly aware of. I have been going to a psychotherapist who works with cancer patients and I have been able to go through a lot of things which have been deeply embedded in me since childhood — resentments and anger. I think this has helped me |

enormously to deal with my illness and whether I get better or not I will feel that something positive has come out of this. I think it is a very important aspect of having cancer. It's the one constant in whatever type of treatment you choose. I don't think there's any treatment myself that would be valid without this psychological factor and I just wondered whether, if you had this facility to call on, you wouldn't even find that your success rate went up?

Dr  I suspect that you're absolutely right. In a way, it is an awful indictment of the manner in which we are able to help our patients. Unfortunately, there is a time factor involved as I have already said; the work keeps coming in and you have to deal with new problems as they arise. In fact, this is an area we are looking at very actively at the moment as we have a nurse psychologist who is passionately interested in patients with cancer. We are anxious to implement a study to examine the psychological aspects of cancer and its treatment, and I think it is very important. Unfortunately, this cannot be done within the NHS as funds are just not available and this will have to be a privately-funded venture.

Diana  If it were set up as a natural part of the treatment to see a psychotherapist people might find it easier to accept; because most people don't regard themselves as psychiatric cases. It's bad enough being told you've got this terrible physical illness without being told that your mind needs sorting out as well. That is obviously a difficult thing, but I suspect that I can't be unique in having felt all these funny emotions. I'm sure it must happen with most people when you're faced with this threat to your life . . .

To me the doctor is the central person. If I decide to go off and do my diet and meditation, etc. and say I'm going to take charge of this, I still like to think you're there in the background if any problem crops up. Even if I don't want it treated, I like to feel that I can consult the doctor to see what is happening.

Dr  It's important to me that you do that. Because I feel very strongly that I don't want to lose touch either.

Rachael  My sense is that, unhappily, this is a very rare situation. On the whole patients who adopt other approaches find that their doctors are not willing to support them or maintain contact.

Dr But you see we are pretty vulnerable people in many ways. We do feel upset if things don't go well, as in your case. We do feel the pressures and an element of this vulnerability is emphasized when someone decides to seek a second opinion elsewhere. You may think: 'God, I'm a failure, I can't do anything right.' Now this can be a very potent reaction, I promise you, particularly if you have become deeply involved and you do care. It highlights the failure thus far of the treatments we have been able to give. I think there are some people involved in your own case who will find it very difficult to come to terms with the fact that you made a decision to seek alternatives and I shall probably get blasted for it. I happen not to have any hang-ups about people seeking other opinions because my view is that this is their right and that if it is going to help them, then that's fine. After all, that's what we're all aiming for and it may be very important for an individual to explore alternative opinions at a particular time. I think it would be awful for you to go away feeling that I was saying: 'OK, that's the cut-off point. If you are not prepared to do what I think then that's it.'

Rachael In most cases it takes enormous courage for patients to question their doctor's treatment.

Dr They don't want to upset their doctors.

Rachael The patient protects the doctor.

Dr Yes, my patients protect me all the time by telling me things they think I wish to hear and not telling me things they think will upset me. They want to please me because I am trying to help them.

Rachael Do you think Diana is representative of an increasing number of patients in their approach to their illness?

Dr Yes, I think she is. I think many more patients go through conventional treatment and also look at alternatives without telling their doctors.

Rachael My sense is that it is the patients who are drawing the doctors out to look at different approaches.

Dr Yes, I think they are. We are conditioned to a certain extent by our training. Certainly my own training was related to the mechanics of diagnosis and treatment of disease. There was very little emphasis placed on the art of communication with patients — what you should tell people and how you should tell them. This was something that was assumed you could pick up by watching your peers at work. In fact, there is a lot that can be taught about this very important area.

Rachael  Diana, as a patient, what do you feel you most need from your doctor?

Diana  I require from my doctor and have actually received in this case professional knowledge and frankness to the extent that I will be involved in decisions about treatment. In my particular case it has involved making decisions not to accept the treatment being offered, but at least I am being given the same information upon which to base my decisions as you have had to make yours. So the purely professional aspect of professional knowledge and laying out of available alternatives is of paramount importance. That is why I come to a doctor. But underneath that, it is nice to have the moral support and to feel that he is expressing some sympathy with the patient having to undergo arduous treatment. And, if the patient does opt for alternatives and he has to go back to the doctor, as I have had to do, to feel that I am not going to be turned aside because I have turned him aside.

Rachael  And what do you need from your patients?

Dr  What I need from my patients is a warm, friendly and sympathetic relationship as well as the understanding that we are in this problem together and that I don't necessarily have all the answers. The input that each individual patient is prepared to give me is very important when I am making a decision, particularly when it is not a black and white one.

There are many situations in which the decision regarding the best form of treatment is very difficult. If I am not able to discuss with the patient how he or she is feeling about the various options, and if he or she simply tries to put all the responsibility onto the doctor, it makes the decision that much more difficult. Therefore, I very much value the contribution of my patients.

Rachael  In summing up, what I hear from you Diana, is that you

|           | want open information, on which you can base your decisions, plus you want genuine human contact. |
|-----------|---|
| Diana     | Yes. |
| Rachael   | And what you are saying, Dr Phillips, is that you want patients to be willing to be responsible, to give you their advice and you want some human contact too. |
| Dr        | Yes. I want much the same from my patients as they want from me. |
| Rachael   | What, if anything, do you think you have gained from each other? |
| Dr        | I have gained a tremendous amount from you, there is no doubt about that. It has been a very warm and open relationship and you have actually made my job much easier because of your understanding and the way you have come to terms with your illness. The way you have coped with all the set-backs has been tremendous. I think that what I have learned from you is that by analysing yourself more closely you have been able to come to terms with what are extremely demoralizing and difficult problems in a quite remarkable way, and really quite quickly too. I know that you feel much more fulfilled as a person and much more at peace with yourself and this has been very gratifying. This whole process has been very important for me because hopefully I might now be able to point others in the same direction. I am not sure how much I can help them directly to do it, and I doubt very much if I helped you to do it. This was largely something that came from within yourself, but it was very important for me to have seen it. |
| Diana     | Well, I think that because we have had this very warm human relationship, it has emphasized the human side of the illness for me. I think the fact that my relationship with my doctor has not been purely clinical, in the sense of being able to discuss other aspects of my illness with you, and to feel that I was being listened to with sympathy and interest, has helped me. It certainly helped me through the rigours of the treatment. I have felt a very great need to talk to you. |
| Dr        | And I you. You see, it is a two-way process. |
| Diana     | Yes, I have felt this need to express my feelings and to know that although you might only have been treating |

the physical aspects of the illness you understood the emotional concepts in which they were there.

I think it has been a very warm and revealing experience, because I feel that I now understand doctors much more and I understand the doctor's point of view and the context within which medical advice and decisions are taken. I think I have a much greater understanding and respect for the medical profession now, as a result of knowing you, then I had before. Not because all doctors behave like you, but because most doctors must feel and think like you. Because you have been prepared to reveal to me how your mind works, how you approach clinical decisions, your feelings about a patient, I therefore realize that although other doctors may not always reveal it, nevertheless they feel it.

You're quite right when you say about patients protecting doctors, because when I think about our discussions the other day, I felt very sorry for you having to talk to me like that.

Dr   I think you handled me very beautifully. At the end of the day, I think it is very important that all of us looking after patients do actually care what happens to them as individuals and that we show that we care. If you can do this, it means so much. There are people with whom I work who I'm sure do care, but can't actually communicate it. They are unable or unwilling to let themselves go and allow people to realize that it does matter to them if things go right or wrong.

Diana   One of the things is that one is faced with the thought, 'Does it really matter if I go on living, is it worth it?' This is a question I am asking myself constantly and part of the back-up to this is the fact that you can establish human feeling with the people you have contact with and who are specifically involved in your illness. I think just simply feeling this human warmth in a way contributes to wanting to go on living.

**Afterwards**

My sister died aged forty-nine, just three months after this conversation took place. In that time she was able to come to terms with her situation in the same spirit of courage and acceptance that she dealt with her illness. She found great peace and, with the help of healing and the local hospice home-care team, she had no pain. She was able to die at home, where she wanted to be, surrounded by those she loved, including her two children.

She managed to make the trip to the Bristol Centre and stayed for two weeks. That, and the work she did with her psychotherapist, meant a great deal to her and she was able to make peace with her past. She said, 'I've had a life of fulfilment. The fact that I couldn't think of anything else to do and couldn't imagine a future, probably meant that it was time for me to go. I feel my life is whole now and no longer in parts. I've reconciled the past and got rid of all the clutter. I don't have any pain, I feel fine. I just wish everyone could feel as I do.'

I asked her what she felt she'd learned from her life and she replied, 'I've learned that life is continuous and that there's something creative in all of it. I've learned to let go of being responsible for other people and that you can trust them. There's far more to people than I ever imagined.'

When I started this book I little thought that so many of the ideas and suggestions I have made would be tested in such a way. Now they are part of my personal experience. I know that for each person it is different, but the fact that Diana had the courage to take responsibility for her illness, and that she strove to learn and understand herself, helped her enormously. Through it she was able to give so much to those around her — we all grew.

It was easy to support her and respond to her strength and frankness. Her openness and humour helped us to come to terms with the situation. Because we were able to nurse her at home, although this was arduous at times, we felt the better for being with her and helping her. I cannot speak highly enough of Trinity Hospice home-care team. Their care and love was genuine and expert. As it happened, we did conduct the funeral service ourselves and it was indeed helpful. We were able, through poetry and other pieces, to express our feelings for Diana far better than any stranger could have. Over two hundred people were present and I know that many of their lives will not be the same for having been there.

Diana had no fear of dying and was able to joke about it without any sense of denial. Her main concern was for people around her. She sought ways to ease their distress and find them comfort. She had scores of visitors from home and abroad and was able to complete all her relationships, expressing appreciation for their friendship.

She hoped that by dying peacefully, and without fear, she might help those who did fear death. She certainly did so and bequeathed a great gift to us all.

It is ironic that I should know two such different people, both with cancer. Their stories have different endings and yet there's much in common. Thankfully Roger lives on in good health, but both achieved fulfilment through their illness. Because of it they have inspired many others and I am proud to have known them both.

# 10.

# WHERE TO GET HELP

Throughout this book I have indicated various sources of help and support. While it is true that nobody can do it all for you, it is equally true that you cannot do it entirely alone. In dealing with a major life crisis such as cancer, it is surprising the number of people who, in different ways, help us to get through.

When I think of my own situation and those close to me, the number of people who have supported us in some way must run to well over a hundred. Whether it is the good neighbour who helps with the shopping, or the good wishes and healing thoughts of friends and acquaintances, they all combine to build a network of support. When Roger was ill, there were even groups of people regularly praying for him in different parts of the country. My sister, too, was overwhelmed by the love and good wishes coming to her from people she had never met.

Whether it is a healing conversation with the hospital cleaner or the expertise of the doctors and nursing staff, they are all part of your team. Social workers, information exchanged with the patient in the next bed, books, counsellors, self-help groups, children, friends and family all provide pieces in the jigsaw.

You have something to offer too, in sharing your experience you may be a link in someone else's network. A large proportion of those involved with helping others, including myself, have come to do so only because their lives have been touched by personal experience of cancer. You may not know it but you are also a teacher; it is *only* through you that the doctors, healers and researchers are learning to combat the disease we call cancer. Each one of us is a link in that chain as we seek to resolve our own predicament.

## Cancer Support Groups

Self-help groups have in recent years become an increasingly valuable part of any support network. As people come to receive they also find something to offer. The act of giving can be a powerful therapy for anyone who feels diminished by their circumstances. As well as providing for those who have a particular problem self-help groups create a much-needed link between the lay people and the professional carers. They help to voice and bring about changes, by giving feedback to experts who think they know all about cancer, but who have never stood in the shoes of those they care for. Modern health care usually ends at the hospital gate and it is often when treatment finishes that people need support in coping with their situation.

It is really only in the last few years that cancer support groups have begun to be established in this country. In 1982, when Roger and I first thought about setting one up, we were astounded to find only a handful scattered throughout the country and none in London. Now local groups are springing up everywhere and national or regional network organizations, providing back-up facilities, have been established.

CARE (Cancer Aftercare and Rehabilitation Society), and CancerLink are two of these. CancerLink was started in 1982 by four people who contacted each other after a television programme on cancer. Three had been professionally involved in cancer research and education and two of the four had been cancer patients themselves. CancerLink provides expert medical back-up, advice and training courses for cancer support group volunteers. It also has a national information service.

British Association of Cancer United Patients (BACUP) is another national organization giving advice and information to cancer patients. It also offers a counselling service and publishes booklets. BACUP was started by a doctor who was a cancer patient and is medically based.

New Approaches to Cancer provides a network and forum for those interested in complementary therapies. There are now many cancer support groups which focus on this type of approach. The Bristol Cancer Help Centre is, in itself, a major support system where patients using their methods attend on a monthly basis.

Like any organization, many of these networks have had their teething problems, but they broke ground in creating a way for patients and volunteers to support each other through the experience of cancer.

At first there was much opposition from the medical profession, who are reluctant to entrust the care of their patients to unqualified people. Perhaps their caution is understandable because cancer patients are, after all, in a highly vulnerable situation and the desire to do good isn't always a criterion for the ability to provide it.

On the other hand, a cancer support group can provide something that most professionals can't — first-hand experience. During the time I was involved with running a group it was overwhelmingly obvious how much people benefited from talking to someone else who had experienced cancer. This is particularly so when people are first diagnosed, when they are still in shock and terrified about what's going to happen to them.

One conversation can make all the difference to that person's ability to handle their illness and treatment. The major reaction is one of relief and reassurance. I also found that people felt it much safer to release their feelings with those who they knew would understand. Many a time people would walk in the door and feel safe enough to just burst into tears. Others felt freer to make difficult choices about treatment; some left with the reassurance to go through with it and others found the courage to refuse.

People often feel they have to live up to some imagined expectation of being a 'good patient'. They may be afraid that their carers will be less caring if they step out of line. The roles of doctor/authority and patient/victim which we tend to adopt, can make it difficult for open communication.

However well a doctor or nurse tries to explain what it will be like to have an operation or treatment, there is nothing like talking to someone who has had it. It is important to remember though, that one person's experience may not be the same as another's. This is particularly so with cancer, and is another reason why health professionals have been so reluctant to approve of patients getting together. Anyone running a group needs to bear this in mind and be aware of some of the situations which could arise.

One person's cancer may be more treatable than another's and bringing them together may raise false hopes or even false fears. Even those with the same diagnosis may not get on well as people. Whilst finding 'someone like you' is helpful, overdependency can present difficulties. If someone bases their confidence on the progress of another, it may be shaken if that person has a recurrence.

Overdependency on the group also has to be considered.

People who become over-attached to being a permanent patient, dwelling only in the world of cancer and sickness, may be best encouraged to let go of cancer and involve themselves in other activities.

Respect for the person's chosen way of dealing with their illness is of prime importance. Organizers or group members may have strongly-held beliefs or opinions about a particular approach to treatment. While motives may be of the best, it is easy to end up imposing your way on someone else.

Whilst running a cancer support group certainly has its demands, it also has tremendous rewards. All in all, cancer support groups provide a necessary service, not only for members, but also for the community at large by dispelling fear and alienation. For many people merely meeting a cancer patient is a major confrontation. I have seen people walk into a meeting expecting to see wasted cripples in wheelchairs, people with no hair, and finding themselves amazed to see a bunch of normal-looking joyful people.

Cancer patients often have to deal with the added pressure of being seen as a freak by family and friends. The group provides a setting where they are able to be themselves again and share their experience without overconcern for the reaction of others.

One of the things which struck me most forcibly about the group was the atmosphere of love, friendship and aliveness. I was aware of the people more than their situations. Sometimes the social events were the most creative — the tea-breaks at meetings, where people made individual contact and swopped information; the jumble sale where everyone enjoyed being able to give and participate.

When we are ill, we so often lapse into helplessness and depression. Giving reminds us that we are people not illnesses and that we are still capable of rising above our circumstances. One girl, a leukaemia patient, raised nearly three hundred pounds by doing a sponsored swim which she organized herself. Another woman, who died shortly after a bone marrow transplant, spent her last weeks in the special isolation unit, writing fund-raising letters to celebrities and giving books to other patients and staff.

Of course, a group setting doesn't suit everybody. Many feel nervous or restricted when with a number of people. Others just do not relish the idea of any kind of organized activity. A large number of people are still afraid to admit that they have cancer and even contacting a group at all requires a lot of courage. Most groups do however provide a telephone counselling and information service, or home visits, as well as meetings.

Some feel that associating with other cancer patients works against their approach to creating a positive will. For them it overemphasizes the aspect of cancer and illness. Their way is to try and forget about seeing themselves as a cancer patient and to remember as much as possible that they are a normal human being with a situation to resolve.

Whatever your point of view, it is useful to know that help and support is available if and when you need it. Whether you are a patient or a supporter, you need not cope alone.

> I lived on the shady side of the
> road and watched my neighbours'
> gardens across the way, revelling
> in the sunshine.
>
> I felt I was poor, and from door
> to door, went with my hunger.
>
> The more they gave me from
> their careless abundance the
> more I became aware of my beggar's bowl
>
> Till one morning I awoke from my sleep
> at the sudden opening of my door, and
> you came and asked for alms.
>
> In despair I broke open the lid of my
> chest and was startled into finding my own wealth.
>
> Rabindranath Tagore

# Appendix

# SETTING UP A SUPPORT GROUP

If you are sufficiently recovered from treatment and you are interested in setting up a local group, here are some basic guidelines which you may find useful.

### A. Local Contacts
Start by finding out what services are already available. In doing so you will also make contacts which may be useful to you. Contact your District Health Authority, Social Services Department, local Council for Voluntary Service, Community Health Council, Community Centres and hospital Social Services Department.

### B. Forming a Core Group of Volunteers
1. You can advertise through various means; cards in shop windows, letters or interviews with local newspapers and radio. *Be specific that you want people who are interested and able to give help,* otherwise you may receive requests for help instead.

2. It is advisable to see people individually before arranging a meeting. Sometimes people want to give help but may be more in need of help which you are not yet ready to provide.

3. Arrange a meeting for prospective volunteers. It is helpful to take plenty of time to get to know each other and form your ideas about what kind of service you want and are able to provide. It is important to have a core group who know each other well and who are clear about how much each is able and prepared to give.

4. It is essential that the core group is well supported; that the group doesn't become dependent on one person and the load

is spread. In any group there is tendency for the same few willing people to end up doing all the work. It works well to have at least three or four people in the core group and to make sure that members participate as much as possible. One way is to set limits about what you are prepared to do for the group. You can select roles, with one person in charge of a specific area. One person, for example, might like to act as librarian, collecting and organizing a library of leaflets, books and other useful information. Another might like to be in charge of arranging meetings and guest speakers, etc.

5. *It is vital to have a proportion of people in good health.* Problems can arise if key volunteers frequently have to go into hospital. In fact you may want to establish some criterion of fitness for all active volunteers. This could be based on the length of time since a person has finished their treatment.

6. Forming a committee is necessary if you are going to handle or raise money. If you are receiving public funds, it will also be necessary to form a constitution which sets out the aims, structure and membership rules of your group. Committees should have a chairperson, secretary, treasurer and other members.

7. You may decide to become a charity, this has financial benefits as well as giving an air of respectability to a group when approaching others for money. Forming a charity can be complicated and you may find it far simpler to associate yourself with one of the umbrella organizations previously mentioned. You will then have the benefit of their charity status without the rigmarole of setting one up.

If however, you decide to be independent, the National Council for Voluntary Organizations (26 Bedford Square, London, WC1) has a legal department which can handle this for you, free of charge. Interaction Inprint publish a book called *Charitable Status, a Practical Handbook* (available by post, from Interaction Inprint, 15 Wilkin Street, London NW5 3NG, price £4.50). This book is a 'must' for anyone trying to understand the intricacies and definitions of charity law.

8. You may wish to involve one or two professionals on your committee. This can of course be a valuable contribution but remember that a support group is essentially run by and for people with cancer and their relatives. It is a place where people learn that their own experience is a source of strength and support

# SETTING UP A SUPPORT GROUP

for themselves and others. Professionals are also frequently busy with little time to spare for committee work. However, they may be more than willing to act in an advisory way.

## C. Receiving Requests for Help, Meetings, etc.

Any local form of advertising can be a way to let people know about your group.

Local contacts already mentioned, plus local churches may help you find a meeting place. Day centres are sometimes available, although not always free of charge. It is important when selecting a venue to bear in mind ease of access. This applies both to transport and to those members who might not be fully mobile; in other words, not too many stairs.

It may be possible to get free printing, photocopying or even use of typewriters through your local contacts. Friendly local businesses may also be willing to help out.

Before giving out publicity about the group, which may involve listing private telephone numbers, think about how volunteers will cope with phone calls coming to their home. One solution is to get a separate line for the group with an answer-phone, so the person whose home it is can have times when they don't need to answer calls.

## D. Useful Guidelines in Talking to People with Cancer

The golden rule is to help people in the way they wish to be supported, rather than imposing on them your own opinions about what they should or shouldn't do.

With over a hundred types of cancer, each person's diagnosis and response to treatment will be different. Patients may be frightened about their own chances of recovery because they have heard about someone else's bad experience.

It is good practice to admit when you 'don't know'. You can always find out who might know and refer people on if necessary. It is important to set limits about the extent of information you can give. You will be acting primarily as a friend, someone who understands through personal experience.

# USEFUL ADDRESSES

**United Kingdom**

1. National Organizations
Carers National Association
29 Chilworth Mews, London
W2 3RG
Tel: (01) 724 7776
Offers support to relatives, the chronically ill or disabled. Gives practical advice plus contacts for local self-help groups.

British Association of Cancer United Patients (BACUP)
121-123 Charterhouse Street, London EC1M 6AA
Tel: (01) 608 1785/6
Runs advice and information service for cancer patients and their families and friends.

British Red Cross Society
9 Grosvenor Crescent, London SW1X 7EJ
Tel: (01) 235 5454
Will loan practical items for the use of home care. Some local branches provide volunteers to sit in with patients while supporting relative and friends have a break.

Health Education Authority
Hamilton House, Mabledon Place, London WC1H 9TX
Tel: (01) 631 0930
Publishes a source list of cancer education publications and teaching aids.

## USEFUL ADDRESSES

Help for Health
The Grant Building, Southampton General Hospital, Southampton SO9 4XY Tel: (0703) 777222
Offers a written and telephone information service. They have also published a guide to books written from personal experience (see Recommended Reading).

The Leukaemia Research Fund
43 Great Ormond Street, London WC1N 3JJ
Tel: (01) 405 0101
Although their prime function is research, they also publish some useful information leaflets on leukaemia, Hodgkin's disease and other lymphomas.

The Marie Curie Memorial Foundation
28 Belgrave Square, London SW1X 8QG
Tel: (01) 235 3325
This organization is involved with research and education as well as patient care. They offer advice and counselling to patients and relatives. They also have eleven Marie Curie Homes providing short to long stay terminal care facilities. In addition they offer a nationwide home nursing service for terminal patients, arranged through local communiites.

Cancer Relief Macmillan Fund
Anchor House, 15/19 Britten Street, London SW3 3TZ
Tel: (01) 351 7811
Provides financial assistance for cancer sufferers in need. Small grants are available to help pay for any heavy personal debts, extra heating, hospital travel for patients and relatives, home nursing and convalescence. Applications are made via local authority or hospital social services departments. They have recently developed the Macmillan Service which provides specially trained nurses for terminal home care as well as a small number of Macmillan Units. Macmillan Units provide hospice type facilities all on hospital sites and run by the NHS.

Tenovus Cancer Information Centre
142 Whitchurch Road, Cardiff CF4 3JN
Tel: (0222) 619846
Publishes a range of leaflets and operates a telephone counselling and information service.

## 2. Specific Types of Cancer

**Chest, Heart and Stroke Association**
Tavistock House, Tavistock Square, London WC1H 9JE
Tel: (01) 387 3012
Gives financial aid and counselling to people with lung cancer.

**British Colostomy Association**
38/39 Eccleston Square, London SW1V 1PB
Tel: (01) 828 5175
Offers advice and information in adjusting to living with a colostomy. They have a national network of branches with trained volunteers who counsel patients at home or in hospital. All volunteers have had a colostomy.

**The Ileostomy Association**
Amblehurst House, Chobham, Woking, Surrey GU24 8PZ
Tel: (09905) 8277
Runs a similar service for ileostomy patients.

**The Kingston Trust**
The Drove, Kempshott, Basingstoke, Hants RG22 5LU
Tel: (0256) 52320
Runs convalescent/rehabilitation homes in Essex and West Yorkshire for all stoma patients.

**The Breast Care and Mastectomy Association**
26a Harrison Street (off Grays Inn Road), Kings Cross,
London WC1H 9JG
Tel: (01) 837 0908
Gives information and advice on all aspects of breast cancer from early detection and breast self-examination, to practical information about prostheses and suitable clothing. Through their network of local branches, volunteer counsellors visit patients both before and after their operation. All volunteers have themselves had a mastectomy.

**The National Association of Laryngectomy Clubs**
4th Floor, 39 Eccleston Square, London SW1V 1PB
Tel: (01) 834 2857
Has clubs throughout the country to support people who have had a laryngectomy. They offer speech-therapy, social support and meet monthly. They also visit patients before and after their operation.

Society for the Prevention of Asbestosis and Industrial Diseases (SPAID)
38 Drapers Road, Enfield, Middlesex EN2 8LU
Tel: (0707) 873025
Gives information about claims, inquest procedures and DHSS benefits.

The Urinary Conduit Association
8 Conniston Close, Dane Bank, Denton, Manchester M34 2EU
Tel: (061) 336 8818
Operates a similar service to other stoma organizations for ureostomy patients.

The Women's National Cancer Control Campaign
1 South Audley Street, London W1Y 5DQ
Tel: (01) 499 7532/3 (Screening Helpline: (01) 495 4995)
Provides information and advice on early detection of breast and cervical cancer. Also offers help and advice to women who may have or who are being treated for cancer.

### 3. Childhood Cancer
Cancer and Leukaemia in Childhood Trust (CLIC)
Pembroke House, 11 Fremantle Square, Cotham, Bristol
Tel: (0272) 248844
Gives support and financial aid to parents. Owns a holiday home in Devon, plus two houses in the West Country offering accommodation to parents while their children are in hospital.

The Family Fund
PO Box 50, York YO1 1UY
Tel: (0904) 621115
Offers financial help to families of chronically sick children. Also help with practical items, e.g. bedding, clothing, etc.

The Leukaemia Care Society
PO Box 82, Exeter, Devon EX2 5DP
Tel: (0392) 218514
Provides mutual support contacts for families of child or *adult* sufferers. Also organizes caravan holidays and can give financial aid.

The Malcolm Sargent Cancer Fund for Children
14 Abingdon Road, London W8 6AF
Can provide cash grants to parents of children under the age of twenty-one. Applications should be made via a hospital social worker.

National Association for the Welfare of Children in Hospital
Argyle House, 29-31 Euston Road, London, NW1 2SD
Tel: (01) 833 2041
Gives practical and social support as well as advice and information to sick children and their families.

### 4. Sexual Problems
Sexual and Personal Relationships for People with a Disability
286 Camden Road, London N7 0BJ
Tel: (01) 607 8851/2
Advice, information and referral service for the disabled.

Marriage Guidance Council
76a New Cavendish Street, Harley Street, London W1M 7LB
Tel: (01) 580 1087
Gives counselling individually and jointly. Contact for local branch.

Family Planning Information Service
27/35 Mortimer Street, London W1N 7RJ
Tel: (01) 636 7866
Will refer people to individual counsellors nationwide.

### 5. Hospice Care and Bereavement
Macmillan Units and Nurses (see Cancer Relief Macmillan Fund, page 142).

Marie Curie Foundation (page 142).

Age Concern
Bernard Sunley House, 60 Pitcairn Road, Mitcham, Surrey
Tel: (01) 640 5431
Operates numerous services for the elderly through local branches. Also provides bereavement counselling.

Hospice Information Service
St. Christopher's Hospice, Lawrie Park Road, Sydenham,
London SE26 6D7
Tel: (01) 778 9252
Provides a directory of hospice and other in-patient care, as well as home-care teams and hospital support teams throughout the UK and Eire.

The Sue Ryder Foundation
Cavendish, Sudbury, Suffolk CO10 8AY
Tel: (0787) 280252
Runs homes for people with cancer.

Compassionate Friends
6 Denmark Street, Bristol BS1 5DQ
Tel: (0272) 292778
Offers mutual self-help and counselling contacts for bereaved parents.

CRUSE
Cruse House, 126 Sheen Road, Richmond, Surrey TW9 1UR
Tel: (01) 940 4818/9047
Has a network of local branches offering counselling and practical advice to the bereaved and their children.

Friends of Shanti Nilaya
Old Cherry Orchard, Forest Row, East Sussex
Aims to provide support based on the work of Dr Elisabeth Kübler Ross.

## 6. Cancer Support Groups (Networks)

Cancer Aftercare and Rehabilitation Society (CARE)
21 Zetland Road, Bristol BS6 7AH
Tel: (0272) 427419
Has a number of independently-run associate groups throughout the country.

CancerLink
17 Britannia Street, London WC1X 9JN
Tel: (01) 833 2451
Has several local groups in SE England. Also has a national telephone information and counselling service and provides a

directory of all cancer support groups throughout the UK. Runs a counselling skills training course for cancer support group volunteers.

Serious Physical Illness
The William Kyle Centre, 23 Kensington Square, London W8 5HN
Tel: (01) 937 6956

Coping with Cancer Northumbria
3 Cottenham Street, Westgate Hill, Newcastle Upon Tyne
Tel: (0632) 732064
Parent body for Coping with Cancer Groups in NE England.

Tak Tent
132 Hill Street, Glasgow G3
Tel: (041) 332 3639
Counselling and information, plus contacts for Scotland.

## 7. Complementary Approaches

New Approaches to Cancer
c/o The Seekers Trust, 8a The Close, Addington Park,
Nr Maidstone, Kent ME19 5BL
Tel: (0206) 860874
Offers information and advice about all aspects of complementary therapies. Has a directory of practitioners, centres and cancer support groups interested in this approach. Promotes conferences and events with international speakers.

The Bristol Cancer Help Centre
Grove House, Cornwallis Grove, Bristol BS8 4PG
Tel: (0272) 743216
Offers in-patient and support facilities on a monthly visiting basis. Provides a list of affiliated support groups and practitioners.

The British Holistic Medical Association
129 Gloucester Place, London NW1 6DX
Tel: (01) 262 5299
Education and information service. Provides a list of medical practitioners interested in the holistic approach.

Centre for Attitudinal Healing (SE only)
PO Box 2023 London W12 9NY
Tel: (01) 235 6733/200 7155/549 2529
Support groups and one-to-one counselling for anyone faced with serious illness. The work is non-medical and complementary to existing treatment. There is a commitment to help each other achieve a shift in perception from fear to love which facilitates attitudinal healing.

## 8. Specific Therapies

Community Health Foundation
188 Old Street, London EC1V 9BP
Tel: (01) 251 4076
For those interested in macrobiotics.

British Acupuncture Association
34 Alderney Street, London SW1V 4EU
Registry of practitioners.

Traditional Acupuncture Society
11 Grange Park, Stratford-upon-Avon, Warwickshire CV37 6XH

Association for Therapeutic Healers
Write c/o Celia McNab, 'Derbyshire', Crank Road,
Kings Moss, St Helens, Lancs.
Tel: (01) 240 0176
A small but growing organization for those who combine healing with other therapies (eg. psychotherapy, biofeedback, etc.)

The Confederation of Healing Organisations
c/o Dennis Haviland, 113 Hampstead Way, London NW11 7JN
Umbrella organization with contacts for the whole country.

National Federation of Spiritual Healers (NFSH)
Church Street, Sunbury-on-Thames, Middlesex TW16 6RG'
Tel: (0932) 783164
Has a list of member healers throughout the country.

British Homoeopathic Association
27a Devonshire Street, London W1 1RJ
Tel: (01) 935 2163
Provides a list of medically qualified practitioners and hospitals.

Society of Homoeopaths
101 Sebastian Avenue, Shenfield, Brentwood, Essex CM15 8PP
Has a register of non-medically qualified professional practitioners.

Association of Hypnotists and Psychotherapists
12 Cross Street, Nelson, Lancs BB9 7EN
Tel: (0282) 699378
Provides a nationwide practitioner list.

For psychotherapists using the transpersonal approach:
Trust for the Furtherance of Psychosynthesis and Education
188 Old St, London EC1
Tel: (01) 608 2231

Institute of Psychosynthesis
310 Finchley Road, London NW3
Tel: (01) 486 2588

## 9. International Contacts
World Cancer Care Federation
28 Belgrave Square, London SW1
Tel: (01) 235 3325
Gives information on all contacts worldwide.

**USA**

The American Cancer Society
777 Third Avenue, New York, New York 10017
Tel: (212) 371 2900
For information and local contacts.

Cancer Care Inc. of the National Cancer Foundation
Cancer Care Inc, One Park Ave., New York, New York 10016
Tel: (212) 679 5700
Voluntary agency providing professional counselling and advice.

Candlelighters Foundation
123 C. St. SE, Washington DC 20003
Tel: (202) 483 9100/544 1696
National organization for parents of children with cancer.

# USEFUL ADDRESSES

Cancer Counselling and Research Centre
1300 Summit Ave., Suite 710, Fort Worth, Texas
Centre based on the work of Carl and Stephanie Simonton

Can Surmount
American Cancer Society, 777 Third Ave., New York, New York, New York 10017
Provides volunteer support to patients and families. Referrals through the patient's doctor.

Centre for Attitudinal Healing
19 Main Street, Tiberon, California, 94920
Tel: (415) 435 5022
Centre for children faced with life-threatening illnesses. Support for families and siblings of the patient. Based on the work of Dr Gerry Jampolsky. Other centres exist throughout the USA, contact this address for details.

Leukaemia Society of America Inc.
211 East 42nd Street, New York, New York 10017
Tel: (212) 573 8484
Provides financial aid and information to leukaemia, Hodgkin's disease and lymphoma patients.

Make Today Count
PO Box 303, Burlington, Iowa 52601
This is a self-help group for people with incurable diseases, their families and professional carers.

The National Hospice Organization
Tower Suits 506, 301 Maple Ave., West, Vienna, Virginia 22180
Gives information about hospice care nationwide.

Shanti Nilaya
PO Box 2396, Escondido, California
Centre founded by Elizabeth Kübler Ross. Holds regular workshops for the dying, their families and health professionals.

United Ostomy Association
111 Wilshire Boulevard, Los Angeles, California 90017
Tel: (213) 481 2811
Offers emotional and practical support to patients with stomas.

## Canada

Canadian Cancer Society
National Office, Suite 1001, 130 Bloor St. West, Toronto,
Ontario M5S 2VS
Tel: (416) 961 7223

Victoria Hospice
Royal Jubilee Hospital, Victoria General Hospital, 1900 Fort Street,
Victoria, British Columbia V8X 1B9.

## Australia

Australian Cancer Society
Box 4708, Sydney, NSW 2001
Tel: (02) 231 3355

ACT Cancer Society
PO Box 135, Civic Square, ACT, Australia 2608

Cancer Council of Western Australia
705 Murray Street, Perth, Western Australia 6000

Silver Chain Nursing Association (Continuing Care)
19 Wright Street, Perth, Western Australia 6000

## New Zealand

Cancer Society of New Zealand
The Secretary, Box 10340, Wellington

Hospice care contacts:
Dr Graeme Campbell, FRACP, FRCP, Consultant Physician,
St. Joseph's Hospice, Mater Hospital, Auckland, New Zealand.
Dr Richard Turnbull, Medical Director, Te Omanga Hospice,
PO 30814, Lower Hutt, New Zealand

# RECOMMENDED READING

Here is a selection of the increasing number of books available on the market. I have included those which I have read myself and some particularly recommended to me as being useful and relevant to the reader. I have also included titles already mentioned throughout this book.

**General Information**
*The Cancer Reference Book*, Paul M. Levitt and Elissa S. Guralnick (Harper and Row, 1984).
*All About Cancer*, Chris Williams (John Wiley & Sons, 1983).
Both books are medically informative but contain aspects which some patients may find offputting.

**Specific Types of Cancer**
*Breast Cancer*, Caroline Faulder (Virago Press, 1982).
*Breast Cancer — The Facts*, M. Baum (Oxford University Press, 1984).

**Booklets**
General Information Pack — Women's National Cancer Control Campaign (concentrates on early detection. See Useful Addresses for details).
*Living With The Loss of a Breast*, Mastectomy Association and Health Education Council (see Useful Addresses).
*Understanding Colostomy* and *Understanding Ureostomy* both published by Squibb Surgicare (a drug company).
*Back on Your Feet Again*, Colourplast (surgical appliance company).
All these booklets should be available through your GP or hospital.

### Childhood Cancer
*Children With Cancer*, Merren Parker and David Mauger (Cassell Ltd., 1979).

### Relatives and Friends
*The Healing Family*, Stephanie Matthews-Simonton (Bantam Books, 1984).
*How Can I Help?*, Ram Dass & Paul Gorman (Rider, 1986). Emotional Support and spiritual inspiration for those who care for others.

### Practical Information
*Guide for The Disabled Traveller*, published by the Automobile Association. Provides a comprehensive list of holiday accommodation, with details of facilities.

### Personality and Stress Related to Cancer, also Attitudinal Healing
*Getting Well Again*, Carl and Stephanie Simonton (Bantam Books, 1978).
*You Can Fight for Your Life*, Lawrence Le Shan (Thorsons, 1984). (The emotional factors in the treatment of cancer).
Both of these books are excellent in highlighting the personality aspects of cancer.
*Love is Letting Go of Fear*, Gerald G. Jampolsky (Bantam Books, 1982).
*Teach Only Love*, Gerald G. Jampolsky (Bantam Books, 1984).
*I Want One Thing*, Francis Horne (De Vorss and Co., 1981). With specific chapter entitled 'Towards Transformation Through Cancer'.

### Complementary Approaches
*Holistic Health*, Lawrence Le Shan (Thorsons, 1984). A brilliant summary of the current revolution in health-attitudes and how to use them.
*The Gate of Healing*, Dr Ian Pearce (Spearman, 1983).
*The Bristol Diet*, Dr Alec Forbes (Century, 1984).
*The Cancer Prevention Diet*, Michio Kushi (Thorsons, 1984). For those interested in macrobiotics.
*Healing*, edited by Lorna St Aubyn (Heinemann, 1983).
*New Approaches to Cancer*, Shirley Harrison (Century, 1987).
*Love, Medicine And Miracles*, Bernie Segal (Century, 1988).

## Death, Bereavement and Hospice Care

*On Death and Dying*, Dr Elisabeth Kübler Ross (Tavistock Press, 1977).
*Death the Final Stage of Growth*, Dr Elisabeth Kübler Ross (Prentice Hall Inc., 1975).
*Who Dies?*, Stephen Levine (Anchor Doubleday, 1982).
*Grist for the Mill*, Ram Dass (Wildwood House Ltd., 1978).
*The Courage to Grieve*, Judith Tatelbaum (Heinemann, 1984).
*Hospice, A Living Idea*, ed Cicily Saunders (Edward Anrold, 1981).
*The Hospice Alternative*, Margaret Manning (Souvenir Press, 1984).
*Dying at Home*, Harriet Copperman (John Wiley & Sons, 1983).
*A Reckoning*, May Sarton (Women's Press, 1984). A fictional account of a woman dying of cancer.

## Personal Experiences

*Champion's Story*, Bob Champion and Jonathan Powell (Victor Gollancz, 1981). Autobiographical account of the English jockey's successful fight against testicular cancer.
*A Way To Die*, Rosemary and Victor Zorza (Andre Deutsch, 1980). Parents' account of their daughter and her experience of melanoma. Includes a frank description of her dying and of her final stay in a hospice.
*One Day at a Time*, Pat Seed (Pan Books, 1979). Written by a woman journalist who went on to campaign for funds to provide scanning equipment, before dying of cancer in 1984.
*A Gentle Way With Cancer*, Brenda Kidman (Century, 1984). Written by a woman who chose to use alternative methods of treatment after being diagnosed with breast cancer.
*Fighting for Our Lives*, Kit Mouat (Heretic Books, 1984). A collection of personal accounts gathered by the author, who now runs a self-help organization called Cancer Contact. Focuses on the use of homoeopathy in treating cancer.
*Reflections*, Bob Gann (available by post from Wessex and Regional Library and Information Service. See Help for Health for address details). Guide to autobiographical books written by people faced with serious illness. There is a section on cancer listing a range of books and giving reviews of each one.
*The Cancer Journals*, Audre Lorde (Sheba Feminist Publishers, 1985). A fiercely passionate account of the author's experience of facing breast cancer and mastectomy. Argues the moral issues surrounding prothesis i.e. she sees it as a way of denying the experience for all concerned.

# GLOSSARY

**Acupuncture** — An ancient Chinese system of medicine which uses ultra-fine needles to stimulate subtle energy points in the body. It can be used to treat the physical, emotional or mental level of a person.
**Adjunctive treatment** — Treatment which is additional to the main course of treatment e.g. after breast surgery, radiotherapy is often used as an adjunctive treatment to insure the eradication of any stray cells.
**Allopathic medicine** — Medicine based on the treatment and eradication of symptoms.
**Benign** — Non-cancerous.
**Biofeedback** — A self-training technique which teaches people to recognize and control their own stress and relaxation responses.
**Biopsy** — A microscopic sample of suspect body tissue from which diagnosis is made.
**Carcinogen** — Cancer producing substances which are found in the environment. They may be natural or man-made e.g. tobacco tar, radiation.
**Carcinoma** — Cancers which develop in the lining layers of organs, the digestive system and the skin.
**CAT scan** — A sophisticated X-ray technique which enables a three-dimensional picture to be built up.
**Chemotherapy** — Intense drug treatment which destroys all fast dividing cells, primarily the cancerous ones.
**Choriocarcinoma** — Cancer of the placenta in pregnancy.
**Cytotoxic** — Poisonous to cells.
**Domiciliary care** — Care which takes place in the person's home.
**Hodgkin's disease** — Cancer of the lymph system, more commonly found in young people.
**Holistic** — Perceiving life from the point of view of the whole rather than the parts. In medicine, treating the whole person body, mind and spirit as one inseparable organism.
**Homoeopathy** — A drugless therapy based on the principle of immunization which uses natural remedies to stimulate the person's natural self-healing ability.

# GLOSSARY

**Implants** — Small radioactive objects which are placed inside the body close to a tumour in order to destroy it.
**Letting go** — Releasing emotional attachment to a situation. It does not mean getting rid of the situation.
**Leukaemia** — Cancer of the blood (there are several types).
**Lymphangiogram** — A test to detect the spread of cancer through the lymph system.
**Lymphatic system** — A system of ductless glands which help to cleanse the body and fight infection.
**Lymphocytes** — Lymph cells.
**Lymphoma** — Cancer of the lymphatic system.
**Lumpectomy** — Removal of a suspicious lump by surgery.
**Macrobiotic** — A dietary system based on the Chinese philosophy of yin and yang and applied to foods.
**Malignant** — Cancerous.
**Mammography** — Breast X-ray.
**Mastectomy** — Removal of the breast (part or whole) by surgery.
**Melanoma** — A skin cancer which develops from malignant growth in a mole.
**Mesothelioma** — A type of lung cancer which develops from contact with asbestos.
**Metasteses** — Secondary tumours seeded from cells that have spread from the original or primary site.
**Monoclonal antibodies** (magic bullets) — Artificially produced substances which can select and destroy cancer cells only.
**MRI** (magnetic resonance imaging) — A type of scan.
**Oncology** — The study of cancer.
**Organic** — Food that is grown without the use of chemical fertilizers or pesticides.
**Orthodox** — Generally accepted or approved. Conventional medicine.
**Palliative** — Pain-relieving.
**Prognosis** — Medical opinion regarding the outcome of a person's treatment or illness.
**Prostate gland** — A gland found in men adjacent to the bladder.
**Radiology** — X-ray photography.
**Radiotherapy** — Treatment of cancer with a series of controlled doses of radiation.
**Relaxation** — A state of consciousness which affects us physically, emotionally and mentally. A peaceful state of being.
**Remission** — When there is no cancer present in the body (not necessarily cure).
**Responsibility** — The act of owning something which gives us the *ability to respond* to life's situations. Not blame.
**Sarcoma** — Cancers which arise in the bone, cartilage or muscle.
**Secondaries** — See metasteses.
**Staging** — Assessment of how far the disease has progressed.

**Stoma** — Diversion of a section of the bowel or urethra to the body surface through surgical means. An external bag is then worn to dispose of bodily waste.

**Terminal care** — Care of the dying.

**Teratoma** — Cancer of the testicle. Found more frequently in young men.

**Transformation** — A major shift in our way of being, a contextual shift which affects every area of our life.

**Transpersonal** — That which is beyond the personal. Our universal sense of self.

**Visualization** — Deliberate and focused use of the imagination to effect mental, emotional or physical change.

**Wholefood** — Unprocessed food, but not necessarily organic.

# INDEX

active participation in treatment, 121-3
acupuncture, 56, 57, 71
alternative therapy, doctors' reac- reactions, 120-21, 126-7

barium meals/enemas, 34
benign tumours, 19
bereavement
  cancer trigger, connection, 26
  facing, 95-6
  incompletion problems, 103-5
biofeedback training, 67-8
biopsy, 34
blood tests, 35
bone secondaries, 20
bowel, cancer of, 20, 23
breast, cancer of, 20, 23, 29
  lumpectomy, 37
  mastectomy, 37
  prosthesis, 33

carcinogens, 23-4
carcinoma, 20
carers, time off, 94-5
case histories, 26, 29-30, 49-51, 85-6, 88-9, 110-116
CAT scans, 35
causes, 21-7
cells and DNA, 19
cervix, cancer of, 25, 29
  laser therapy, 39
chemotherapy, 39-41
children
  with cancer, 96-7
  sharing situation with, 51
choriocarcinoma, 28
complementary approaches, 56-74
conversation, patient/doctor, 117-30
coping and morale, 53-5

counselling, 52-3, 70-71, 93, 96, 104
CT scans, see CAT scans
cures, 27-8
cysts, 19

death, 98-109
  Diana's experience, 130-32
diagnosis, 34-6
  patients' responses, 45-55 107, 117-20
diary-keeping, as therapy, 49
diet
  anti-cancer, 63-6
  cancer link, 23-4, 33
  for radiotherapy and chemotherapy patients, 33, 42-3
differentiation therapy, 43-4
doctors, guide, 31-2
drawing, as therapy, 49

emotional stages, 102-3
environment, causative factor, 22-4
exercise, 79

family
  sharing situation with, 51-2
  their experiences, 90-7
finance, 53
five emotional stages, 102-3
friends
  sharing situation with, 51-2
  their experiences, 90-9

goal setting, 78
grieving process, 104

healing, 72
herbalism, 56
herpes virus, 25
Hodgkin's disease, 20, 28

holistic approaches, 56-74
homoeopathy, 56, 65-6
hospices, 105-6

identity, 107-9
immune system, 25-6, 34
implants, 39
information seeking, 53-4, 91
intravenous pyelogram (IVP), 34

judgement, and positive thinking, 81-3

laser therapy, 39
leukaemia, 20, 28, 35, 40
life transformation, cancer as catalyst, 87-9
life events, 25-7, 50, 103
lumpectomy, 37
lung cancer, 20, 22
lymphangiogram, 34
lymphatic system, 34
lymphomas, 20

macrobiotics (diet), 63-4
magic bullets, 42
magnetic resonance imaging (MRI), 35
malignant tumours, 19
'markers', 35-6
mastectomy, 37
meditation, 67, 79
melanoma, 23, 26
mesothelioma, 22
metastases, 20
monoclonal antibodies, 42

negative thoughts, 81-3
nurses, guide, 33

oncogenes, 24
oncostain, 24
osteopathy, 56
ovaries, cancer of, 25

Pill, cancer link, 21, 22
play, 79-80
'Pool of Forgiveness, The', 82-3
positive thinking, 75-83
predisposition, hereditary, 27

prostate gland, cancer of, 20, 25
prosthesis, 33
psychotherapy, 70-71, 125-6, 131

questions, strategy, 46-7

radiology, 34
radiotherapy, 36, 37-9
relaxation, 58, 67, 67-70, 78-9
remission and partial remission, 28
responsibility, 83-7

sarcoma, 20
scans, 34-5
secondary tumours, 20
self-help methods, 26
self-preservation (saying 'no', letting go of 'shoulds'), 80-83
side-effects, 38, 40-41
skin cancer, 23, 26, 28, 36
smoking, 22, 110-12
spirituality, 72-3
staging, 34
stoma-care, 33
stress, 25-7, 78
  release techniques, 66-70
support groups, 52, 94, 134-7
  setting up, 139-41
surgery, 37
symptoms, 28-9

terminal care, 105-7
testicular cancer, 28, 36, 40
transformation of life, cancer as catalyst, 87-9
treatment, 36-44
tumours, 19

ultrasound scans, 35
uterus, cancer of, 20

visualization, 26, 58, 67, 67-70
vitamin A, 44
vitamin C, 64

warning signs, 28-9

X-rays, 34

yin and yang, 58-9, 64